Annemarie Goldstein Jutel

DIAGNOSIS

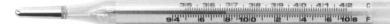

TRUTHS
AND
TALES

With Thierry Jutel and Ian Williams
Foreword by Lisa Sanders, MD

UNIVERSITY OF TORONTO PRESS

Toronto Buffalo London

ISBN 978-1-4875-0302-4 (cloth)
ISBN 978-1-4875-2226-1 (paper)

Printed on acid-free paper with vegetable-based inks.

Library and Archives Canada Cataloguing in Publication

Jutel, Annemarie, author
Diagnosis : truths and tales / Annemarie Goldstein Jutel ;
with Thierry Jutel and Ian Williams ; foreword by Lisa Sanders, MD.

Includes bibliographical references and index.
ISBN 978-1-4875-0302-4 (cloth). ISBN 978-1-4875-2226-1 (paper)

1. Social medicine. 2 . Diagnosis – Social aspects.
3. Diagnosis – Psychological aspects. 4. Popular culture. I. Title.

RA418.J88 2019   362.1   C2018-906309-2

Thermometer image used for editorial break: bluebright/iStock

University of Toronto Press acknowledges the financial assistance to its
publishing program of the Canada Council for the Arts and the Ontario Arts
Council, an agency of the Government of Ontario.

 Canada Council
for the Arts
Conseil des Arts
du Canada

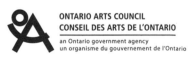 ONTARIO ARTS COUNCIL
CONSEIL DES ARTS DE L'ONTARIO
an Ontario government agency
un organisme du gouvernement de l'Ontario

Funded by the   Financé par le
Government   gouvernement
of Canada   du Canada
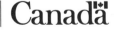 Canadä

To Lydia Wevers for her support, her example, and her friendship.

Contents

Illustrations

Foreword:
Giving the Story Back

The medical encounter is, fundamentally, the creation and exchange of stories between patient and doctor.

It goes something like this: The patient experiences something – we can call it a symptom – and develops his own story about that experience. That story may include elements such as where he was or what he was doing when the symptom began; what it felt like; what he thought of it; and why he chose to seek medical attention. He may then bring that story to his physician. She may then add to it with additional questions and possibly a physical examination; she may order some tests and include those results. It is the physician's job to then reshape that story and give it a name, a title, a diagnosis. She may even add a glimpse into the next chapter – the treatment and prognosis.

Having created a new edition of this patient's story, the physician must give that story back to her patient and to do it in a way that allows him to try it on and, if it seems to fit, to incorporate this new version of his story back into the bigger story of his life.

As physicians, most of what we learn focuses on the first part of that process: how to add to the patient's story, how to reshape it, and how to rename it. We get all kinds of training in making the diagnosis, and in treating the disease captured within the diagnosis, but this whole business of giving it back was for years relegated to the "art" part of medicine and until recently wasn't even taught to doctors. And yet it is one of the most important parts of our job. Done well, the patient has a sense of what is happening to them, what is going to happen to them, and what can be done.

And we do this all the time. As Jutel acknowledges, when we take something we've experienced to a doctor, we expect a diagnosis. We demand a diagnosis. It seems natural and inevitable. A patient comes in with a fever and sore throat, cough, and body aches during flu season. We swab the back of their throat to confirm what we already suspect – this is the flu – and give them a prescription for Tamiflu. It's an almost invisible transfer of the story from patient to doctor back to patient. But there are other stories that are harder to give back, harder to tell. And those are the stories we never forget.

In my second year of training, I reviewed the chart of a 55-year-old man I'd never met but was supposed to see in clinic at the end of the day. He was a patient of one of my fellow residents and was coming to get the results of a recent CT scan. An unusual reason for an appointment, I thought, until I read the radiologist's report. It was bad. A large mass in the head of the pancreas. So large it was partially blocking the upper part of the intestines. Other masses were seen in the liver as well. The diagnosis was suggested by the radiologist: Pancreatic cancer that had spread to the liver. A biopsy was needed to confirm it. My job, as I could see it, was to let him know that this was probably a malignancy and get him to both the cancer surgeon and the oncologist.

I considered what I'd been taught about breaking this kind of news. We'd had a lecture on it in med school:

First you find out what the patient knows.

Then you give a hint that the news you have isn't good.

Then you tell them what you know.

Then you address their feelings.

Then you get them to see the specialist.

Five steps. Easy.

Because I'd never met this patient, I wasn't at all sure what to expect. From reading his chart, I could see that he was a guy who didn't see the doctor often. His thin chart carried only his insurance information and notes on the two visits he'd had with my colleague the week before. He'd come to see a doctor because he was vomiting any time he ate anything. They tried medicines and when that didn't work, he had the CT scan. And now he was coming back.

He was the last patient on my schedule, and I was grateful. Breaking this kind of news, I thought, could take a while. I had the patient's chart in my hand as I entered the small exam room. I introduced myself to the patient and his wife and sat down. The patient was very thin and moved restlessly in his chair as we spoke. The mild jaundice from the way this mass blocked the liver made him look suntanned, though there was still snow on the ground. His eyes were nervous, darting. His shirt hung loosely from his thin frame and I could see he'd lost a lot of weight. "Tell me what you understand about what's going on," I said, trying to keep my tone level.

"It's cancer. It's cancer." He jumped up and strode to the window. Turning to look at his wife, he exclaimed, "I told you, it's cancer. If it was anything else they wouldn't have told us to come here today." He glared at me, "I mean, why couldn't you just tell me over the phone?"

Not going the way I expected.

"So hang on," I tried. "Let's not get ahead of ourselves," I said, my voice cracking.

"It's the liver, right, doc?" he turned to his wife. "I told you." Then he turned back to me, "How long do I have?"

"There was a mass seen on the CT scan," I tried again to frame this story in a way that allowed the possibility of hope, of next steps.

Cancer, right?

I tried to explain that a diagnosis wasn't possible based on the CT alone but that was certainly a possibility. The next step was for him to see a surgeon and an oncologist, and I had already made the referrals and had the phone numbers.

"More doctors?" he asked, as if I had suggested some crazy course of action. "I think I've seen enough doctors. Let's go." He motioned to his wife. "I told you this would be a waste of time." He strode out of the room. His wife gathered her coat and purse and followed. I trailed behind trying to slow him down, to have the conversation I'd rehearsed in my head. Near the door he turned to me, "Look lady, I don't want any of this." He waved his hand indicating the exam rooms and clinic. "If I'm dying, I sure ain't doing it here. And if I'm not, no offence but what do I need you for?" And with that he put his arm around his wife and strode out.

It's been 15 years since I met that patient. Though he is long dead by now, I suspect, he lives on vividly in my memory. I've replayed this encounter countless times. Certainly, I could have handled it better. And the set-up was clearly a problem. He'd been stewing about this since he had received the call to come in.

We think of the diagnosis story as our story, the doctor's story. The patient has the symptoms, the questions, but we have the answer, the diagnosis. But, actually, it is never really our story. It is always his story. In this case, it was a story he'd shared reluctantly. And in the end, he decided to take it back. I don't know how much we might have done to change his prognosis. I'd like to think that, at the very least, we could have made the remainder of his life a little better. But that's not how he wanted his story to end.

In the years since the afternoon of that terrible education, I have seen countless patients, received their stories, done what I could with them, and given them back, as best I could. And yet, for the most part, this leg of the story, this transfer of the story from doctor back to patient, remains murky territory.

Thus, this volume, dedicated to the exploration of that murky territory, is a welcome addition to the scholarship and to understanding diagnosis. The stories I describe above – the patient story before and after and the doctors version in between – are not the only stories at play. These stories have been shaped by other stories: there are those we were taught in school; those we heard others tell before us; those we watch in the news on TV or read in novels or biographies. The stories of diagnosis are everywhere. And they are important. These stories have power to shape how we think, how we feel, how we act. And they have the power to shape the world around us: how we are seen, how we are understood, and how we are remembered. Indeed, the diagnostic story can have power that far exceeds the concrete reality beneath – the actual disease that prompted the story in the first place. The diagnostic story can reveal important aspects about medicine and health, but in *Diagnosis: Truths and Tales* Jutel demonstrates that these stories reveal even more about the world we live in, the roles we inhabit, and the creation and transformation of identity.

This examination of how the doctor and patient see, shape, and understand their respective stories is an important and untold aspect of medicine and society. And long overdue.

Lisa Sanders, MD, FACP

Acknowledgments

Many people have helped me to write *Diagnosis: Truths and Tales*. Thanks are in order first to Thierry Jutel and Ian Williams for contributing chapters to this work, and to Lisa Sanders for writing the foreword, but more importantly, for helping me to think more broadly about the subject. For research support, I thank the splendid library staff at the Center for the History of Medicine at the Harvard Countway Library and at the Wellcome Collection in London. Justin Cargill at the Victoria University Library gets a special mention for his continuous support. Many people have read also and commented on the work in various stages of production. I thank my colleagues who have read my work and given me critical feedback: Douglas Booth, Anna Jackson, and Joanna Kempner, and the anonymous reviewers.

And as always, thanks to Ellen Goldstein, champion wordsmith.

DIAGNOSIS: TRUTHS AND TALES

Introduction

Imagine the following scene. You've had a series of physical symptoms, none of them terribly serious on their own, but together adding up to a slightly worrisome total. You've gone to the doctor, who agreed that a diagnostic workup was in order. You've had an X-ray, maybe a scan, and some blood work. The results are back, and you are in the doctor's office, awaiting the verdict. On the one hand, you're thinking, It's probably nothing. I've just been overworked recently. On the other, you are wondering, Suppose it's something serious?

Maybe you are a doctor. This is the kind of scene you run through in your head as well. It's sometimes your job to deliver difficult information about disease. You've done the diagnostic workup. You've taken the patient's sometimes-rambling story and poked and prodded it into shape. You've thought hard about what might be ailing her, and now with the labs and scans in hand, you are about to tell her. It's going to be hard, this moment of truth.

We have probably all rehearsed this kind of scene in our heads. What would we do/say/think/feel if the doctor were to say, "I'm sorry to have to tell you this, but you have [name of dire diagnosis]." We might have a list of activities to tick off, people with whom to reconcile, places to see, or things to do. The announcement of a serious diagnosis is a solemn moment, when directions shift, priorities change, and life appears in sharper focus.

The doctor too is rehearsing. In this one moment, with just a few short words, the doctor can overturn a patient's sense of themselves and the doctor knows it. He or she will be thinking about how the information can best be delivered, will hearken back to a previous case or a previous patient, or a faraway med school mentor whom they held in high esteem and imagine how that person might approach this difficult moment.

The naming of a serious diagnosis is a powerful thing. It changes how we think about our bodies, our disorders, our futures, and even our identities. The naming of the disease can sometimes be more powerful than the disease itself. The doctor's words, as Schofield wrote at the turn of the last century, have "double force"[1] at a moment like this.

The *disease* itself, of course, influences our experience of life. It brings our awareness of our bodies forward in our consciousness. Rather than being the tool by which we explore our world, and reach out for our fulfilment, the sick body complains, creaks, and disobeys our intentions. Instead of fading into the background, as we act on our goals and engage our desires, it is constantly surfacing to remind us of its dysfunction.[2] But the power of the *diagnosis* is something different.

The diagnostic moment imposes an indelible boundary on life, dividing "a life into 'before' and 'after,' ... [a division] ... henceforth superimposed onto every rewrite of the individual's life story," according to Suzanne Fleischman, a linguist whose own life was thus cleaved when she learned she had what was to be a fatal leukaemia.[3]

The moment a diagnosis is named, even if that moment is not quite as circumscribed as in the scene I depict above, is a moment in which a story is told. It is a story we are able to imagine, even if we haven't experienced or witnessed it before, because the diagnosis is so common a device in stories of all kinds. Diagnosis is, in itself, a story. It links together a set of phenomena in a usually linear manner; it generates an explanation, a plot line, and a denouement in which a knotted bundle of threads gets untangled. It *represents* disease, in the sense that it presents the inside world of disease to an external audience (one which includes the patient) using words, stereotypes and motifs that are immediately recognizable.[4]

The stories of diagnosis are told in a particular tone, with an expectation of a particular kind of outcome. This is why we can imagine the diagnostic scene. We've seen it in before in many other guises: a sombre newspaper report about a celebrity learning about an unexpected cancer, a book in which the protagonist must wrestle with the knowledge of his newly announced disease, a film in which the main character watches her life wind down after learning she has an early-onset dementia.

Diagnosis is part of many stories in ways that are immediately recognizable yet sometimes hidden. Diagnosis is frequently the key to a story, and to a character's trajectory or identity, but it is often woven into the tapestry so seamlessly that the reader barely notices it. It is structurally embedded in how we tell stories, yet not visible. It needs calling out. That this moment is so common, that we take it in stride, without even seeing it, is the important issue that this book confronts. Diagnosis is as pervasive in popular media as it is in medicine, part of a particular kind of storytelling that shapes how we meet these difficult experiences of, and conversations about, disease.

Throughout this book, and via numerous media, I will reveal the stories triggered by diagnosis and consider the way they shape our social, and individual, thinking about a moment like the one that opened this Introduction. I will expose the narrative nature of diagnosis and reveal how its discursive construction as truth instils it with various forms of power: transformative, authoritative, and administrative.

Every serious diagnosis sets loose a multitude of stories. From the stories conceived of, told, and retold by the patient quietly to herself before she goes to the doctor, to the story the doctor carefully prepares and rehearses before delivering it to the patient, and to the many stories that will be told afterwards by the patient, the doctor, and their respective entourages, diagnosis is at their core. The diagnostic moment serves as a poignant stimulus for these stories and many more in our lives. *Diagnosis: Truths and Tales* explores stories about diagnosis and ponders the impact they have on how we experience health and disease.

The stories associated with diagnosis, and particularly about the moment a diagnosis is offered to a patient, are interesting because they are so prevalent, so influential, yet at the same time, so invisible. They are told by doctors, sick people, well people, novelists, film-makers, and advertisers. They appear in books, on film, on the radio, online, and, well ... almost everywhere!

I wrote this book both to render visible and to defuse these influential stories. The rendering visible, the revelation, is not just for the purpose of detailing their frequency and pointing to their occurrences. More importantly, it is to demonstrate their influence. As I will expose in the chapters that follow, and as I described above, they are powerful social tools, these stories. They shape how we think about health, illness, and disease. They structure authority in our society and determine who gets access to resources. They force us to look at our identity and our futures in ways we might otherwise take for granted.

There are many ways to discuss and explain these stories, but my discussion will be framed by intersecting and overlapping perspectives. I cannot restrict myself to a historical analysis or a sociological one. But neither will I position this book in medical humanities or in literary criticism. Placing the analysis in one or in another silo would do little to expand our thinking about the role these stories play.

People in many scholarly disciplines talk about narrative, ranging from literary theorists to philosophers, psychologists, sociologists, and anthropologists. Each discipline has its own way of considering stories. The literary scholar might focus on the structure of narrative, its themes, conventions, and symbols; while the sociologist will be more concerned with the structure or function of a narrative creation.

I prefer to think of the narratives of diagnosis as a version of the "boundary object" as described by Star and Griesemer.[5] These "objects" are positioned at the intersection of what these authors call "different worlds" with different aims and theoretic positions, but with simultaneously shared goals. To explain more simply, these objects are positioned in the middle of a kind of Venn diagram. They belong completely to each set in which they are positioned, different though they may be, and yet at the same time, they belong to all.

The stories of diagnosis are a special kind of object with "multiple memberships."[6] They are examples of how different worlds can share the "same territory."[7] The diagnosis narrative is, in a way, a theoretical boundary object that the critical theorist, literary critic, medical humanity scholar, sociologist, anthropologist, clinician, and patient (only to name a few) can all claim.

To understand how to pull all of these different locations together, or at least see how they interface, Bruno Latour's suggestion about what it is to be a critical scholar is useful here. It is "not the one who debunks, but the one who assembles. The critic is not the one who lifts the rugs from under the feet of the naive believers, but the one who offers the participants arenas in which to gather."[8] There are many arenas in which we can gather to discuss these stories. That is, in fact, the point, and one aspect of the power of the diagnosis narrative. While one camp may see the point of studying the diagnosis narrative as a way of humanizing medicine, of serving its practice,[9] another may see it as a way of denouncing medicine and its reductive stances.[10] These narratives may be cast as pressure valves with therapeutic potential,[11] as vehicles of political activism,[12] as "guidebooks to the medical experience,"[13] and so on. *Diagnosis: Truths and Tales* will assemble the examples and the arenas and propose a way through: one that will alight upon one frame and then another to find alternative ways of narrating a serious diagnosis.

We might commence this reflection on diagnostic stories by pondering classification; diagnosis is a classification tool, and it is via the establishment of disease categories that diagnostic narratives can emerge and where influence starts. Diagnoses are not fixed and static; they are constantly changing in line with advances in technology and social priorities. We should reread the words of Thomas Arnold given to the Rugby Literary and Scientific Society.[14] Writing in the great age of classification when naturalists were developing taxonomies to describe the world, its occupants, its fauna and flora, he observed: "We are not to suppose that there are only a certain number of divisions in any subject, and that unless we follow these, we shall divide it wrongly and unsuccessfully: on the contrary every subject is as it were all joints, it will divide wherever we choose to strike it, and therefore according to our particular object at different times we shall see fit to divide it very differently."[15] While we might take exception to some other of Arnold's positions on education and on the ways of the world, this particular reflection on how classification takes place is nonetheless illuminating. In any case, it certainly reflects a deeply held belief in categorization as a practical and conscious action. The fever tree depicted in figure I.1 is an example of how categories are used to shape thinking. Centuries prior, Socrates had proclaimed that he was a "lover of these processes of division and bringing together, as aids to speech and thought; and if I think any other man is able to see things that can naturally be collected into one and divided into many, him I follow after and 'walk in his footsteps as if he were a god.'"[16]

In diagnosis, medicine (usually doctors) makes the divisions, and this is already a demonstration of how diagnostic narratives convey power, the godliness to which Socrates refers. Diagnosis is, in itself, a process of division. The etymology of the word *diagnosis* is from the Greek. It means to tease out differences, to separate, or to recognize divisions in a subject: from διά (*diá*, "apart") + γιγνώσκειν (*gignōskein*, "to

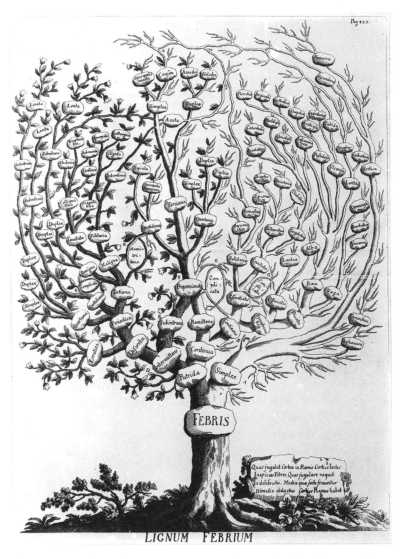

I.1 Diagnosis as clear-cut categories: A Scientific Classification of Fevers. Fever tree. [Illustration from a work by Prof. Torti of Modena University, Therapeutice specialis ad febres periodicas perniciosas, 1712. Credit: Wellcome Collection]

learn"). It was first mentioned in the medical context by Thomas Willis who defined it in his tables as "Dilucidation, or Knowledg" in 1681.[17] By 1701, the Rev George William Lemon referred to "diagnostics" [*qui est dignoscendi, peritus*: subtle discerner]: "A knowledge or judgement of the apparent signs of a distemper, or a skill by which the present condition of a distemper is perceived, and this is three-fold, *viz.* 1. A right judgment of the part affected. 2. Of the disease itself. 3. Of its case."[18] Today, we speak of diagnosis both as the category and as the process by which an individual's ailments are categorized.[19]

As the boundaries are determined, their repeated use then naturalizes them so that we fail to recognize other ways one might choose to strike. The boundaries that circumscribe the diagnosis are drawn with indelible ink, cutting short the debate about where else the lines could be drawn, cementing the disease as The Way Things Are, although, in reality, it is only the way we *say* (think) things are, in a particular context or in a particular point in time. Once the classification system exists, we stop questioning how it got there, since we use the categories to make sense of our world, and as we naturalize these classifications, we fail to consider an important principle. No study of the word *natural* should fail to touch on that other great ideological word, *real.*[20]

For every diagnosis, in addition to whatever natural or biological phenomenon is at its base, there is a political, media, biophysical, and metaphorical frame as well. Framing effects are the ways in which "we generally recognize, define, name and categorize disease states and attribute them to a cause or set of causes."[21] We can see this framing in the presence, for example, of obesity, which on the surface, seems like a straightforward condition, immune to social frames. Yet it has powerful social frames. Plumpness (even extreme) has been, and still is, variably seen as desirable or pathological according to era or culture. This is a diagnosis that has changed its means of assessment over time (from visual assessment of excess adiposity to height and weight scales). Even within standard means of assessment (body mass index or BMI), the cut-off levels to define obesity have changed regularly over time. Obesity is a proxy measure for ill-health – a predictor of poor health outcomes – as opposed to a condition in and of itself. BMI is a population measure, based in epidemiology, that is used on individuals with no regard for ethnicity. All these factors demonstrate how obesity is a fluid, changing medical description of something that is not quite the same from era to era, from person to person, or from country to country, despite the material reality of heavy bodies.[22]

Framing is also a feature of narrative: stories cannot exist without form. In this book, which deals with the diagnosis as a trigger for narrative, revealing its frames is as important as the frames it will create in the narratives it elicits.

The frame in which a disease is named is usually set as a moment of drama, be it in the clinic or a television show. That moment of tension, when the lab results are assembled, already inspected to see how they explain (or don't!) the patient's signs and symptoms, is powerful. The doctor takes a deep breath and gets ready to deliver the "judgment."[23] This moment and its message will be the starting point for stories. There will be the story that the doctor will deliver, which will link all the facts of the disease and reassemble them in a way that makes a particular kind of sense. There will be the story that the patient will tell about what this diagnosis means in her life and those of people around her. There is also the story that is inscribed in the medical records, or the correspondence between clinicians, which will be read and reread by future health professionals, and sometimes by the patient herself, who may be surprised by an alternative narrative.[24]

The instant the diagnosis is delivered, storytelling has commenced, and with it, a particular plot line, with its specific kind of punch, is inscribed. There may be a story of relief, in which previously disorganized pieces suddenly click together like a completed jigsaw to show a picture. Or the diagnosis may generate a story of disarray, when a life planned falls apart, the future dissolves, and the sense of self shifts. Hearing a life-threatening diagnosis, or even having one definitively ruled out, is a crisis moment in the life of the individual.[25]

Of course, that "instant" of diagnosis might also be drawn out and not quite so discrete. Another story preceded it (the one that made the person think they needed to see the doctor). There were hints and clues that could mean different things depending on how they were assembled.[26] A lump on the shin could be part of the story about a clumsy girl, always running in to the dishwasher door, left open by her careless brother, or could alternatively be connected to the lymph nodes, the fatigue, and the fever. When does the story of diagnosis start?

Regardless of whether this moment is succinct or drawn out, it is not surprising that it should trigger narrative. Narrative is the way in which a series of events are communicated to a reader, a listener, or a viewer; just as diagnosis is the way in which a set of discrete and potentially chaotic symptoms are explained to a patient. In narrative, events tend to be linked by causality: one thing happened, and as a result another thing happened, and another and another. But what is important here is that in narrative, events are *represented*. They are assembled and made sense of, then retold in a way that *re-presents* a particular case of the occurrence, using all the skills of storytelling and narrativity (the performance of the story). In diagnosis, the same thing happens. The individual looks backwards and forwards to answer the questions, Why me? And why now? The old rugby injury is brought to the fore to explain the gouty knee, the smoky workplace to explain the obstructive pulmonary disease. By developing a narrative explanation for the unexpected or unwelcome diagnosis, the individual wrests back a modicum of control of the situation.[27]

An effective story is more than a list of happenings. Narratives wrangle with human experience and do much more than simply string events together chronologically.[28] To become a narrative, events must be experienced through a subject. Similarly, a diagnostic taxonomy sans patients serves no purpose. The diagnostic narrative begins precisely because the diagnostic event is experienced in a deeply personal way.

The power of diagnosis to trigger narrative is linked with the power that diagnosis affords medicine in general and the doctor in particular. The pursuit of diagnosis brings the patient to the world of medicine. The ability to diagnose confirms the physician's authority. Indeed, diagnosis is so pivotal to Western medical practice that it is hard to imagine medical care without it. The diagnostic narrative provides an explanation for an ailment, an idea of what the treatment options might (or might not) be, a prognosis, and much more. It assigns responsibility for illness, within medicine and outside. It determines which specialty or sub-specialty can take care of which disorders. It also assigns causation, pointing the finger variably, at the patient for example, for what she ought to have done, or to the gene, the effects of which may be out of the patient's control.

Seeking a diagnosis, then, is the impetus for the sick person to consult the doctor and cements authority at the same time as it reinforces patience and submission. Its special features glue together particular kinds of links and explanations. For example, a diagnosis is a kind of shorthand for multiple signs and symptoms, capturing long case descriptions in just a word or three. The simple modified noun *bacterial pneumonia* evokes chest pain, shortness of breath, fever, crackly breath sounds, and a milky X-ray. It leads to antibiotic treatment, rest, and sick leave. Yet it doesn't reveal the curious (and maybe unrelated) neck pain that was the patient's main concern and incited her to consult, and that was the fulcrum to her presenting story. So while a diagnosis summarizes, it also shortens the story, bringing particular aspects of suffering to the fore and obfuscating or leaving others in the shadow. What doesn't fit into the plotline recedes as the diagnosis becomes the dominant account of the case and of the patient. In the hospital, it's common to hear the patient reduced to a narrative metonymy: the myocardial infarct in Room 25, the pneumonia in Ward 3 …

The careful choice of the diagnosis by the clinician is part of a recognition of the stories that will be generated from this label or that one. For example, the choice of codes, or the manner in which an individual's condition is identified in medical records, say different things about the person, his or her character, and the person's future. Where private insurance dominates medical funding, a diagnosis could be chosen with the individual's future well-being in mind. To say that a patient suffers from *adjustment disorder* (signifying a short-term psychological response to an outside event) explains that she is having a hard time in an otherwise "normal" psyche. In contrast, a "major depressive disorder, recurrent episode" describes a constitutional tendency towards depression, a life-long way of being. Whether the recognition of the stories triggered by the choice of diagnosis is to ensure better insurance coverage or optimism in the patient is immaterial.[29] The point is that the label influences how we see the character, the plot, and the possibilities for resolution.

Diagnoses are sometimes manipulated to enable the much-needed resolution to a troubled story. The doctor might avoid, for example, particular diagnostic explanations in relation to cause of death when suicide takes place. This may enable the deceased a burial in hallowed ground and protect the family from the associated stigma.[30] Or the diagnosis of migraine might be deflected in favour of "tension-type headache" in the records of a student hoping one day to go to flight school, as the US Federal Aviation Authority may consider people with migraines unfit to be pilots. Or the diagnosis might be imposed according to a particular set of dominant values that tell tales about what it is to be white or black, wealthy or poor, and how anxieties about race or status impose particular stories (expectations) of disease.[31]

Stories, therefore, shape diagnostic work but not only in relation to the diagnostic category. They shape understandings of the "sick role," or the way in which having a diagnosis – being "sick" – shapes a different social role for the individual thus designated.[32] The fact of disease gives a kind of permission for the person to stop fulfilling other normative social expectations like going to work or even getting out of bed. On the other hand, the sick role requires the adoption of new social behaviours. The patient must be compliant, following medical orders and investing effort in getting better. The social, cultural, and phenomenological position of the diagnosed individual will influence these expectations and the degree to which he or she fulfils them.

This fact is not lost on anyone who has read Anne Fadiman's *The Spirit Catches You and You Fall Down*.[33] In the riveting pages of her book about a Hmong girl and her family's encounter with American medicine, we learn why their respective views are so apparently irreconcilable. Hmong understandings of epilepsy were so far removed from those of the California medical team looking after this child, that the parents and the medical team could find no common ground upon which to make sense of the young girl's seizures. Medicine couldn't be an answer in a culture that saw epilepsy as a spiritual, rather than a pathophysiological, condition. No translation could make up for the cultural divide, because of the absence of a shared frame of reference.

Ultimately, we shouldn't be surprised. Any social scientist can testify to the importance of understanding cultural worlds to understand (or promote) different outcomes. Almost any disease with unequal distribution or outcomes across genders, cultures, or ethnicities carries a range of narratives and explanations to account for these differences.

Capturing these accounts of contest, inequity, and suffering is paramount to understanding and rectifying the differences.[34] Understanding how people experience illness and death is fundamental to enabling better experiences of health and life, as well as of disease. And finally, listening to the stories that diagnosis triggers should make diagnosis easier to perform, as well as easier to bear.

Many doctors have promoted the importance of narrative in medical encounters and in the improvement of medical education. One nineteenth-century physician opined: "There are many times when it is incumbent on the wise physician to prescribe, not a posset or a purgative, but an essay or a poem."[35] Similarly, Silas Weir Mitchell, a prominent nineteenth-century American neurologist and also a writer of fiction, admonished graduating medical students that "you deal not with the bodies of men alone; woe to them and to you if this be your definition of medicine. Men's souls, men's lives, their thoughts, passions and temptations, their secrets and crimes, come all within the range of your experience." As a remedy, he advised that "the best literature of prose and verse is what I ask you to make a part of your mental outfit for that profession in which no accomplishment can possibly be wasted."[36] He was also, ironically, the same physician who ordered Charlotte Perkins Gilman, author of *The Yellow Wallpaper* to stop writing.[37] His belief in enforced idleness as a cure for neurasthenia kept Gilman away from her "habit of story-making," lest it "lead to all manner of excited fancies."[38]

Today, "narrative medicine" refers to an approach to medical education and practice that pays particular interest to stories as a way of understanding what ails patients and achieving better outcomes for them. It is, according to Rita Charon, "a clinical practice informed by the theory and practice of reading, writing, telling and receiving of stories."[39] Narrative medicine brings in another way of looking at patient accounts which otherwise driven by data, evidence, science, disease, and sharp-edged practices which seem to leave the patients forgotten in their wake. Charon describes diagnosis, as I will throughout this book, as a means for emplotment,[40] a way of making sense of a disorganized illness.

Patients, too, have written about the practice of doctors and the experience of being forgotten in the wake. Performing diagnosis transfers power to the diagnostician. Musing on the tension created by this power Anatole Broyard wrote, "I just wish that [my doctor] would *brood* on my situation for perhaps five minutes … as he goes through my flesh, to get at my illness, for each man is ill in his own way … just as he orders blood tests and bone scans … I'd like my doctor to scan *me* to grope for my spirit as well as my prostate."[41] Broyard feels himself transformed at the diagnostic moment from patient *into* diagnosis, a transformation he resists. "I want to be a good story for him," he laments. This is a point that the linguist Fleischmann reflected upon when she described how, in English, we integrate diagnosis into the self, becoming, in some cases, the disease (I *am* diabetic/depressed/schizophrenic). In other cases, we only carry the disease (I *have* pneumonia/lymphoma/cancer).

Broyard doesn't think for a moment that the diagnostician would be anyone other than a doctor, and this is not surprising. The medical jurisdiction over diagnosis is a long-standing source of prestige for doctors. While a number of other professions are gaining some diagnostic privileges (the nurse practitioner, the clinical psychologist, and the physiotherapist also have specific diagnostic realms), their access to diagnostic authority is limited and controlled by medical associations. I will predominantly refer to the traditional doctor-patient dyad in the diagnostic relationship, a decision I made to reflect the dominant role of doctors in the diagnostic process and in the stories that form the basis of this book.

Yet despite these concerns about power, identity, resources, contestation, and who should be entitled to diagnose, I return to my previous statement: it is hard to imagine the practice of contemporary medicine without diagnosis. It is pivotal in providing a sense of direction to both doctor and patient, accompanied as it is with its view of the future (prognosis) and concomitant remedies (treatment). Diagnosis is a rich tool in the explanation and rectification of human suffering. To diagnose or to be diagnosed offers a smidgen of certainty in an uncertain world, connecting various events (symptoms or dysfunction) into a coherent storyline with a resolution (tragic or not) in view.

As I have outlined above, however, the connections and explanations provided by diagnosis are complex and general. No matter how patient-centred the approach to managing them, they remain generalizations. To consider either diagnostic categories or the diagnostic process as a simple pursuit of the truth, available to the assiduous searcher who leaves no stone unturned, is to ignore that complexity and, in the end, to undermine the goals of diagnosis. Diagnosis is only reliably crisp and tidy in the lab, although not always even there. Once released into the clinic – allocated by designated professional groups; received by individuals; linked with resources, social status, health, and even death – diagnosis becomes far messier than anyone (lay or clinician) would hope, a fact that we will discuss in chapter 1.

Regardless of its messiness, we tend to pursue diagnosis vigorously and feel our stories are incomplete or untellable without the diagnosis. When something goes wrong, we want to know what it is, what to call it, how to speak of it, what story it will tell. I referred to the diagnosis as a verdict, a judgment: black and white, non-debatable, a matter of "truth." The diagnosis gives us a sense of certainty and an idea of what way our disorder, disease, or discomfort will evolve. Somewhere, every request for a diagnosis is a kind of request for a story with a happy ending or at least a comprehensible one. The diagnosis can chase away the clouds that worry us when we are feeling poorly. A diagnosis linked to a treatment can reassure us that this is not the end, that we can forge ahead with a life in front of us. On the other hand, a dire diagnosis without hope of cure is devastating. It confirms, indeed, that there won't be a happily ever after (though, as Havi Carel reminds us, even a dire diagnosis is replete with possibility).[42] And so, the diagnostic

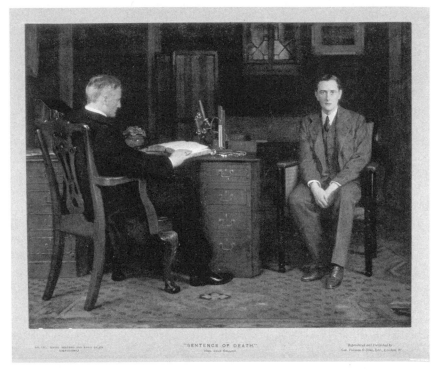

I.2 In the diagnostic moment one story is told and another one is triggered. [Sentence of death. Hon. John Collier. No. 177. Royal Academy and Paris salon. Credit: Wellcome Collection]

moment is one which is filled with suspense. The stakes are high. It is a moment of truth.

As our scene in the doctor's office in the first lines of this Introduction reminds us, diagnosis occupies an important symbolic moment in the spectacle of life and death, the doctor-patient relationship, and interpersonal dynamics. John Collier's painting *Sentence of Death*, depicted in figure I.2, is a powerful example of the awe inspired by the moment of diagnosis. The dramatic and narrative potential of diagnosis also infuses contemporary everyday entertainment. The diagnostic moment is the opening scene in *Breaking Bad*, it was the premise for *The Bucket List*, and the basis for every episode of *House, MD*.

At the same time, the tyranny of diagnosis burdens doctors who have, for centuries, laboured over how to speak of it with their patients, fearful lest they, via their communication, "sound the knell of [the] poor suffering patient."[43] Musings, protocols and admonitions on how to prevent the diagnosis from exercising a "deadly influence ... render[ing] a mild diseases fatal" fill many pages of historical and contemporary publications.[44]

Messy though it may be, diagnosis still matters and matters enormously. How could we make inroads towards either healing or palliation without diagnosis? How could we determine what problems to address, what therapies to test, what outcomes to measure, in the absence of the generalization offered by diagnosis? How diagnosis matters is captured by these generalizations: incidence, distribution, numbers needed to treat. But it is also captured in myriad other stories, the ones that I illuminate in *Diagnosis: Truths and Tales*.

I will take a journey through a range of cultural representations of the diagnosis and its power. I will show how the diagnostic moment is vested with the capacity to define, alter, shift, change, and, ultimately, determine the course of life. This capacity has turned diagnosis into an easily recognizable and recurring device – a trope – for marking a plot, developing a character, or measuring a crisis.

But I will also explore how these tropes return to infuse clinical approaches to the diagnostic moment. I will, of course, critique the power diagnosis is *allowed* to exercise in Western society. The putative certainty associated with this or with that diagnosis is befuddling. People outlive the prognoses associated with their diagnoses and underlive them: they think they are going to succumb to a disease and then get hit by a truck. They fail to respond to the logical treatments associated with a particular diagnosis. The certainty promised by diagnosis is anything but certain. Diagnosis is simply our best attempt at setting some boundaries to health, disease, and life itself.

On this journey, I look at what I have been referring to as *the diagnostic moment* in history, literature, film, and memoir. All these media tell important stories about diagnosis. And, at the same time, each one also provides a different way of understanding diagnosis, in its power and its limitations. These ways matter as much as the biophysical realities of diagnosis and illness, because they identify the ragged edges of the diagnosis and the diagnostic process in ways that taxonomy or classification systems cannot. They help to explain the crises of identity and sources of tension that erupt at or after the diagnostic moment, crises that interfere not only with the lives of patients but also with the work of medicine. They provide, as Martha Stoddard Holmes has written, a way of understanding how we "imagine" our diagnoses even before we receive them.[45]

I have written this book to illustrate how diagnostic narratives recount stories of power and influence. They impose the transformative power of the diagnosis on the patient, the dominance and authority of medicine over the broader public. Stories of diagnosis explain, allocate, and redefine the lives of those diagnosed and of their families. Diagnostic narratives often trump other narratives, replacing, as we said above, previous linkages and explanations. The nature of these narratives and the way in which they distribute power is not unproblematic, and it frequently anchors us in places from which we may want release, whether we be diagnosticians or diagnosees. The book's purpose is to kindle a reflection on what diagnostic narratives do so that we can appraise their impact and consider other formulas for talking about diagnosis. Before we can appropriate them, we must recognize where they are and what they say.

I will focus on some of the important places where diagnosis stories are generated: professional debates between doctors and doctor writings for laypeople, fiction, television and film, graphic art, and illness memoirs. Reading, telling, viewing, and listening to stories about diagnosis, we don't always see the power relations they contain. I will shed a light on these implicit relations of power so that we can reconsider their impact and, possibly, retell these narratives with a better understanding of that impact.

The chapters needn't be read in order, as they can stand alone, and where they don't, I refer to other location in the book. The important characters in the stories of diagnosis are of course the patient, the doctors, and the disease, and each one of these gets its own chapter, even as they wind in and out of the others as well.

I have chosen influenza for my chapter discussing disease, chapter 1. The *flu*, so familiar that we give it a nickname, provides a rich example of how one disease can generate many different and paradoxical stories and exert its status to simultaneously construct and transgress boundaries. It helps to illustrate, as I set out in the opening paragraphs, the limitations of the detective narrative that is so often bestowed upon disease: that a diagnosis is a clear-cut confirmable condition that we hunt out, label, and then treat. Diagnosis is often thought about simplistically, as a label for an unambiguous disorder. Yet diagnoses are often social agreements that reflect values and beliefs more than they are labels. Stories about the common flu help illustrate this and underline the fluidity and the porosity of disease labels. Diagnoses are not as firm as they seem. Telling it like it is is often like it isn't.

Despite this fluidity, patients and doctors alike both pursue diagnosis as the way of making sense of illness. Putting a name to an ailment is an expectation in any illness journey. The process of diagnosis involves defining territory and making claims about truth. We will explore that process in chapter 2, looking at the stories that help get the individual to the doctor's office and are offered up to get the diagnosis going. But we will also consider how patient stories interact with the medical ones, either to enable the medical narrative or to contest it. The narration, or *history*, of a diagnosis can be coauthored, negotiated, surrendered, or withheld by, and between, doctor and patient.

I will describe how authority weaves in and out of the initial stories of illness as they are brought to the doctor for interpretation. We will see how doctors reclaim their sometimes-contested dominance in the storytelling via the creation of a new protagonist, Dr Google, who troubles the traditional roles in the shared storytelling of diagnosis. But I will introduce Dr Google's predecessors, the stories of whom have been around for well over a century. Doctors have been writing for decades about their concerns in relation to free-circulating information about serious medical conditions and how this upsets the layperson and disturbs the doctor-patient relationship. We have, here again, some fabulous stories to unpack from today and from yore, from patients and doctors.

From the patients' stories we will go to the doctors' stories in chapter 3. What doctors say about diagnosis tells us much about what they consider the medical profession to be. I start with historical medical stories – those of nineteenth- and early-twentieth-century doctors – about telling the truth to a patient with a serious disease. This historical departure point provides a fascinating view of how medicine sees diagnosis as empowering the doctor. Hippocrates's words on this subject are probably the earliest we remember. He maintained that "if [the doctor] is able to tell his patients when he visits them not only about their past and present symptoms, but also to tell them what is going to happen, as well as to fill in the details they have omitted, he will increase his reputation as a medical practitioner and people will have no qualms in putting themselves under his care."[46]

Through the stories doctors tell about revealing serious diagnoses to their patients, I will pursue the line prompted by Hippocrates, that is to say, to consider how pronouncing the diagnosis has been connected with professional status and power. These stories, and the characterizations they make of the role of doctors, their patients. and the disease, tell us much about the profession of medicine. We can learn about how doctors see themselves and the place that diagnostic knowledge played, and continues to play, in maintaining their status.

I will show how the doctors' stories about diagnosis characterize the doctors as more than clinicians. The doctor-as-discloser in these narratives becomes, by virtue of the diagnostic announcement, a purveyor of truth, an esoteric professional, a non-lay and non-quack – even a gatekeeper to heaven! It is not only the doctor's knowledge of diagnosis and disease which convey these extra functions but also the manner in which he or she narrates the diagnosis. Words are a "scalpel," wrote Reiser, and therefore a tool to be used judiciously and with training.[47]

Building on this historical work, I will incorporate the voices of contemporary medical writers, pointing out how views of medicine have changed but also what beliefs and values have stayed the same. Doctors' writings are taking pride of place in the popular press. Focusing on the current rise of the doctor-authored trade books on disease, I will examine the stories that these doctor-storytellers write about the diagnostic moment and how this shapes diagnosis today.

What does a doctor write when attempting to convey a sense of his or her work to non-doctors? While the doctor-memoir is a genre on the rise, it is not new; there have been books for a wide public by doctors for centuries. Brown's wrote *Health: Five Lay Sermons to Working People in 1862*, and Hadra followed suit in 1902 with *The Public and the Doctor; By a Regular Physician*. Between, previously, and since these two, books by doctors have attempted to help explain to the layperson what it means to be a doctor. Diagnosis stories feature broadly in these accounts; Hadra explained that "diagnosis is the climax of medical skill and in the profession, no one stands in higher esteem than he who is known to be a fine diagnostician."[48] For that particular section, I draw on the work of Lisa Sanders's (also the author of the foreword to this book) *Every Patient Tells a Story*, Siddartha Mukherjee's *The Emperor of All Maladies*, and Ranjana Svivastava's *Tell Me the Truth* as exemplars.

Following on from these stories by doctors, chapter 4 looks at stories that circulate in the non-specialized setting of the wider public. I will shine a light on popular culture to reveal how the diagnostic moment operates as a trigger or a frame for narrative and for characterization in literature and, in so doing, helps to construct and reinforce its power in medicine. Just as a diagnosis serves to explain illness, prescribe a treatment, and predict outcomes, diagnosis also slots in as an explanatory or transformative device in contemporary fiction. Be it a novel, crime thriller, or short story, many literary forms use the diagnostic moment to set the scene, trigger narratives, explain or resolve a problem, or frame a story. I focus on the analysis of four popular literary works to illustrate the power of the diagnosis in the crafting of fiction.

Using Arthur Hailey's classic *The Final Diagnosis*, we will see how the power to diagnose mirrors power relationships in a local hospital, with every new twist, turn, or stake being linked to a diagnosis, its discovery, or its disclosure. In Anna Funder's *All That I Am*, the diagnosis of Alzheimer's disease opens up rather than shuts down long-gone memories of a traumatic past. It collapses time and provides a frame for the fictional memoire and commemoration of a daring war-time Nazi resistant.

I show how a diagnosis of brain cancer in Michael Morpurgo's *Alone on the Wide, Wide Sea* gives the narrator a starting point for his story by providing him with an end. Morpurgo's protagonist begins: "They say you can't begin a story without knowing the end. Until recently I didn't know the end, but now I do. So I can begin, and I'll begin from the very first day I can be sure I remember."[49] He is a World War II orphan from Britain who sails off to Australia, leaving behind a sister he thinks he can remember. With the end of his life in sight, by virtue of his diagnosis, he hopes to recover his past by penning his memories.

And finally, I explore the magical realism of *The Tiger's Wife* where the power to diagnose bounces the reader back and forth between revelation and secret, certainty and oblivion, duty and destiny. Interwoven in the analysis and discussion of these examples, I introduce numerous other works, such as *Helsinki White, Saturday, The Children's Act, Wednesday the Rabbi Got Wet* (and many more!), to demonstrate the frequency with which diagnosis infiltrates contemporary literature and how it directs, controls, twists, or allocates power, driving the a plot towards its conclusion.

After the chapter on fiction, chapter 5 explores how the diagnostic moment infiltrates television and cinema. The opening scene of the television series *Breaking Bad*, for example, is one of Walter White first being buzzed into an MRI machine then being told of his inoperable lung cancer. He "breaks bad" in reply, transforming his oppressive and dull existence into one of excitement and violence, becoming a drug lord, initially to pay for his treatment, but ultimately to throw off the shackles of his mundane and unhappy life. Working with Thierry Jutel, I will show how the diagnostic moment is represented in TV and cinema and how its transformative potential is used as a device to construct narrative, to drive plot, and to generate character development. From television and mainstream cinema such as Hollywood's *Still Alice* and *Angels over America,* to art house films like *Cléo de 5 à 7* and *The Dallas Buyers' Club*, the diagnostic moment and its impacts on power, social relations, and emotions provide the ingredients to reproduce, question or explore an understanding of health, life, and death.

We demonstrate how the disclosure of a diagnosis and the characters' fictional negotiation of the moment are transformational devices which propel these films and television shows. A character is defined or redefined in the dramatic revelation of a disease that now has a name and requires the character to understand, respond to, and digest the moment. This revelation is an intense dramatic moment that may reveal the character or the stakes as much as it reveals the disease.

The same holds true in other visual forms, and chapter 6 provides a short graphic interlude, with an extract from Ian Williams's *The Bad Doctor*, a graphic novel about the tribulations of medicine, being a doctor, and, of course, diagnosis. The chapter focuses on Julie, a patient who discovers, by accident, that she had previously been given the diagnosis of borderline personality disorder, unbeknown to her. She only discovers upon making an application for life insurance. While the cartoon will incite us to both laugh and sigh at Julie's plight, the short exegesis following these pages will highlight the critical aspects of diagnosis which allow the story captured in this comic to resonate. Without the shared understanding of diagnosis and its function, there would be nothing to smile at. And we can't overlook the fact that this graphic chapter is written by a doctor. In one sense, this is as much about being a doctor as it is about being a patient. The realization of what this doctor can unleash by his simple erasure of her diagnosis is daunting to him. I will also give a brief overview of the emerging field of graphic medicine, which explores the medium of comics and the discourse of health care.

We move from this graphic version of the patient experience to chapter 7, which covers patient tales of being given a serious diagnosis. Particularly in the era of self-publishing, the illness narrative, the patient experience of disease, has become a particularly prevalent form of expression. It serves many functions, from expressive release – a kind of "cry of the flesh"[50] – to self-help and self-redemption, identity making, and exoneration. I look at a particular sub-genre of the illness narrative, what Suzanne Fleischman referred to as the "intellectual documentary" where the philosopher, the linguist, or the creative writer reveals his or her diagnostic moment and how the diagnosis of a life-threatening illness shapes a sense of self and of that person's potential. How do patients learn about, and respond to, the naming of disease? What power do they afford it, and what do they claw back? How does the diagnostic moment, disruptive though it may be, provide at the same time vindication as it legitimizes and validates that the problem as real and worthy of concern?[51]

I tie up *Diagnosis: Truths and Tales* in chapter 8 with a discussion of the potential of narrative to "[provoke] active thinking and [help] us work through problems, even as we tell about them or hear them being told," as H. Porter Abbott wrote.[52] We will pull together the narratives of the previous chapters to reflect upon how we can narrate diagnosis in the clinic. Careful guidelines and doctor training do much to bring to the attention of clinicians the delicate nature of the diagnostic moment, the devastation it can sow, yet they do not highlight or make sense of the range of narratives that explain our expectations of diagnosis.

Importantly, as I highlight the many stories that pervade contemporary and historical popular culture, I must also underline that many other stories are not told and do not hold a place in the popular imaginary. The bulk of the stories I reveal are those of the mainstream. They are the stories of those who can afford to consider medicine as a way of resolving their ailments; those whose stories medicine considers worthy of telling; and those whose stories resonate broadly with a wide public. The stories of the marginalized are rarely told in the same public sphere or with the same influence. The point here is, as it is throughout the book, there are many ways of telling stories about diagnosis, yet popular lore as well as medicine tend to restrict us to a few limited models.

How laypeople of all walks of life experience illness and death is fundamental to promoting change and better experiences of health and life, as well as of disease. A better understanding of diagnosis and its social impact should make diagnosis easier to perform, as well as easier to bear. I conclude by inviting my readers to consider how widely the unwitting use of diagnosis and diagnostic labels infuses understandings of health, illness, disease, and social behaviour. I place an emphasis on both clinical and lay opportunities for discovering new, different, and inclusive narratives for thinking about diagnosis. With diagnosis such an important part of Western medicine, and that position unlikely to change anytime soon, we should consider how the narratives of diagnosis can be told and retold in ways that contribute to, rather than disrupt, our identities, and that reinforce, rather than upset, our lives.

CHAPTER ONE

A Touch of the Flu:
The Paradoxes and
Contradictions of Diagnoses

Influenza gives rise to many stories. What makes it an excellent example with which to start this book is the fact that its stories are so paradoxical and contradictory. On the one hand, flu is depicted as an awe-inspiring disease that has everyone trembling at its ability to decimate populations. On the other hand, it's surprisingly benign: an expected fact of life that inevitably arrives if we forget to get vaccinated (and sometimes even when we remember to!). Flu is a good case study by which to explore how diagnostic stories create intense and potent roles for the disease itself, for those who are infected, and for those who diagnose it. It is also poignant for highlighting how diseases that are characterized as having clear identities often don't.

Flu narratives are pervasive. We read about the flu in the paper, see posters about it on the walls in our workplaces or on the bus, and use the word liberally to describe our ailments. While flu itself is not usually a dire diagnosis, it is a very good example of how diagnosis narratives impose order by the way they are told. They are narratives that create identities, form expectations, and exert a particular shape on our understandings of disease, doctors, and ourselves. Flu narratives, as an exemplar for all diagnoses, also rely upon the idea of scientific truth. The pure objectivity that scientific medicine aims to deliver is based on the notion that diseases are clear and value-free objects that can be captured in diagnostic categories.[1] Flu, a very common physical disease with a known causative agent, however, illustrates just how vague a diagnostic category can be.

Numerous stories feature the flu as a character. It's such a common disorder that just by mentioning it in a sentence, it's as if there were already several paragraphs spoken. Its stereotypical qualities mean that it is recognized in a particular way without having to elaborate. One might refer to "stomach flu"; conjuring up images of all-night vomiting, a lot of time on the toilet, or, at the very least, a queasy loss of appetite. It's a euphemism which describes a garbled-up intestinal tract. We all know, more or less, what it means. This kind of flu has nothing to do with influenza.

Or we might hear about "man flu." The phrase on its own tells a jocular story about a male colleague, deriding him for saying he feels poorly when the general view is he is just not tough enough. Saying "man flu" says as much about the person using the term as it does about the person to whom he or she is referring. It is a kind of wink-wink story that positions a highly gendered narrator as bold, brassy and tough as nails (as well as probably female), and the poor suffering patient as weak, wimpy, and male.[2]

The word *flu* may also be used to describe feeling bad all over, but with an expectation of being well soon. To say someone has the flu could simply be saying that someone has non-specific symptoms that have hit them hard but likely won't kill them. Most of us have heard many stories about fatal flu epidemics, like the one in 1917 that killed an unimaginable number of people. And at the beginning of every winter flu season, the media reminds us about these stories so that this seemingly benign seasonal infection must not be taken lightly. We get regular updates: "Seven people have died in Ireland from flu this season"; "Twenty-four deaths from influenza so far this season, state [Washington] says"; and "*France. La grippe tue 13 résidents d'une maison de retraite*" I read as I went online one day in mid-January.[3]

Flu is an excellent example of how diagnoses themselves give rise to storytelling and how their stories create particular configurations of authority, identity, and entitlement. If classification is based, as we said in the Introduction, on *deciding* where nature should be divided (and by extension what interests are served by a particular classificatory schema), then, the organizational, narrative potential of influenza is particularly salient. I have chosen influenza as the case study for my disease chapter because it is linked to what we think of as a tangible physical disease and yet, despite this, still gives rise to varied, and sometimes paradoxical stories involving shifting boundaries and contradictory accounts. It illustrates how the stories of diagnosis are at the same time familiar and alien, coherent and incompatible. They are about control and about chaos.

I use the terms *influenza* and *flu* quasi-interchangeably as I discuss their stories, even though they are not the same thing. *Flu* (sometimes written with an apostrophe – 'flu – indicating contraction) is the word commonly used to describe a sickness that includes high fever, cough, headache, and sore muscles and often implies infection with influenza virus. These symptoms make up the stereotypical presentation of influenza infection, even though, as we'll see later, there isn't really a stereotype for this wily character! Laypeople and medics alike are inclined to refer to any non-specific, systemic, febrile illness as flu. As a result, the term *flu* tends to capture a range of different kinds of infections, the exact causes of which are generally never known. And yet, doctors, like patients, talk about the flu as if it were influenza. Curiously, barely 20% of people, including doctors and nurses, were able to correctly determine they had influenza, when they used their symptoms as a starting point for diagnosing. More on this later in the chapter.

These stories challenge the ontological nature of diagnosis, because they highlight just how varied and fluid a diagnosis can be. At the same time, these stories locate adjudication and responsibility in different hands at different times. Ironically, these contradictions highlight just how many stories are available for us, and how by retelling, we can provide more opportunities for individuals, nations, and public health.

To observe the complexity and variety of the influenza narratives, we could start by looking back at the not-so-long-ago H1N1 pandemic. The concern about the terrible outcomes we expected (yet didn't receive) reveals countless tensions, controversies, and challenges, all of which are fodder for the stories that arise from diagnosis. The stories were based on two quite contradictory premises. The first casts influenza as a sneaky, nay, treacherous villain. This is the story of influenza's unpredictability and its habit of transgressing any boundary we put in its way. The second, alternative story, however, focuses on the banality of influenza and the shared familiarity that human beings have with its form and consequences. These are distinctly different genres: one a medical/political thriller that keeps the reader perched on the edge of the chair, and the other a G-rated novel, with familiar, domestic themes, predictable outcomes, and no nasty surprises.

Influenza stories that follow the thriller genre hinge on the anxiety introduced by its elusive nature, always infringing boundaries, resisting attempts at its control. Influenza is a slippery virus, hard to pin down in any context, be it etymological, historical, or biophysical. The etymology of the term is French or Italian, depending on which entry of the *Oxford English Dictionary* you consult, and refers to the influence or cause of the disease. In early usage, the disease's name suggested an astral agent, an emanation from the heavens of "an ethereal fluid acting upon the ... destiny of men."[4]

In its history, too, there were countless proposals for its cause. Before microscopy, influenza was not known as infectious. Many other possible explanations were proposed. For example, in 1782, Dr Arthur Broughton suggested influence was due to the "backwardness of the spring, in consequence of which the air has contained a superabundant quantity of phlogiston"; "the action of cold on the surface of the body"; or "the large quantity of rain which fell might cause such a great degree of evaporation from the surface of the earth as to produce a cold sufficient to constringe the pores on the surface of the body, and the great consent between the exhalation from the lungs and the cutaneous perspiration may account for its particular determination to those parts."[5] The influenza described by Broughton was already epidemic, even pandemic. Broughton noted it had made its appearance "in almost every part of Europe and even affect[ing] the inhabitants of America," and he observed that "the symptoms of cough, defluxion, and some degree of fever were characterizing marks of their being affected with what was then termed the fashionable disorder."[6]

Today, however, we usually think of influenza in microbiological terms. *Bacillus influenzae* was brought to our attention in 1892 by bacteriologists Richard Pfeiffer and Shibasaburo Kitasato, who claimed that it was the cause of influenza.[7] They were both correct and mistaken. Although they did assign the cause of influenza in bacteriology, which paved the way for contemporary conceptualization of influenza's causation, they settled on the wrong agent. A virus, not a bacterium, is responsible for influenza.[8] The presence of an easily identifiable causative agent could have contained influenza tidily and made the stories it generated rather straightforward, but for a variety of reasons, the opposite has happened.

First, the influenza virus is constantly in flux via mutation, and even the original identification of the bacillus and, subsequently, the virus were only snapshots of the forms present at the time. Mutation is a viral response to the problem of host immunity. Once exposed to a virus, an individual makes antibodies in response to particular glycoproteins on its surface. These antibodies provide immunity in the presence of a subsequent infection by the same virus. To circumvent this antibody response, the glycoproteins mutate, transforming the virus itself and rendering the antibody response less, or not at all, protective.[9]

Second, new influenza subtypes also emerge from completely new vectors of the disease. The common hypothesis is that they arise from the amalgamation of animal and human strains of influenza. The theory is that a species – usually a bird or a pig – can be infected by both human and animal influenza and experiences simultaneous dual infection. During this episode, the viral material from the animal and human strains is genetically rearranged to result in a novel virus to which most humans have not been previously exposed and are hence susceptible.[10] When the infection can jump from human to human, we have a new influenza strain.

Indeed, the idea of influenza being able to continually reinvent itself gave rise to stories couched in anxiety about the stability of civilization, as the virus travelled from supposedly underdeveloped agrarian nations to threaten the developed West. Actually, the whole idea of classifying disease, and inventing lists of diagnoses to describe these diseases took root in the idea of national boundary protection. The International Classification of Diseases (ICD), developed by the World Health Organization (WHO), with its first rendition published in 1893, was designed as an information-gathering practice by nation states anxious to understand, support, and monitor their citizenry. The genesis of the ICD was in state politics; it was developed in response to nineteenth-century epidemics. The reach of germs had expanded, thanks to the speed and ease of modern travel. The new travel networks ensured that the influenza virus could jump ship at ports across the globe: its victims had more chance of surviving long enough to contaminate a second nation. Classifications therefore had to be able to cross national boundaries along with the germs.[11]

Being able to monitor where any diagnosis jumps ship and re-infects a new pool of unsuspecting victims is part of the "work" an international diagnostic classification document enacts, but also generates numerous public stories about society and what counts as "civilized." The nurse who brings back Ebola from Central Africa, the case 0 for HIV, and the Mexican hacienda where swine flu escaped and headed towards northern borders (more below) all give rise to enthralling tales that glue us to our televisions for the evening news, as, with a frisson, we wonder just how safe our civilization truly is.[12]

Influenza stories, like those of other infectious diseases, are notable precisely because of this sneaky virus's ability to ignore the invisible boundary lines that define nations, terrifying officials and citizens by the way it slips through border control: no passport, no visa. The theme of national boundary transgression is embedded in the notion of pandemic. After all, what is a pandemic but "an epidemic occurring worldwide, or over a very wide area, crossing international boundaries and usually affecting a large number of people"?[13]

With bird flu (the most recent incursion of which arrived five years before swine flu) in 2004, anxiety spread as quickly as the virus. None of the multiple strains of avian influenza experienced by birds usually infects humans, and an epizootic, where only animals are infected, causes less concern. An epidemic – when people are sick – is what gets us worried. In late 2003 and early 2004, outbreaks of bird influenza were also associated with severe human illness, even death, in China, Thailand, and Vietnam. However, with only one possible exception, all cases of infection were restricted to people who worked with birds. There was no obvious human-to-human transmission.[14]

Media narratives about bird flu focused on the depiction of peasant farmers living among their fowl and slaughtering chickens in their backyards.[15] Initially the threat was faraway, in a land where people looked and acted differently from the "civilized" Westerner. But charting of the spread of the virus showed movement from "out there" to "almost here." This tapped existing fears of "Asian invasion," further mixing the idea of immigration with the idea of contagion.[16] Stories about the avian flu used invasion metaphors, usually military: "like enemy troops moving into place for an attack, the bird flu known as A(H5N1) has been steadily advancing," and "Diseases don't stop at state lines, any more than they do at national borders."[17]

In popular imagination, the H1N1 pandemic of 2009 began in a similar way, arising from a rough and muddy hacienda in Mexico where pigs, dogs, humans and other mammals mingled – peacefully, although not, one imagined, sanitarily. However, what really happened was that cases of a swine-origin influenza A were simultaneously described in Mexico and in Southern California in early April.[18] It is possible that the disease started in a brick rancher in San Diego, rather than in a Mexican hacienda, a fact overlooked by the media. The story of a Mexican threat had more purchase.

Couching the origin of the threat south of the border was important to a pre-existing narrative by anti-immigration lobbyists and the conservative media in the United States who were quick to try to attach H1N1 to the much-maligned Mexican migration.[19] However, although Congress could alter immigration law, there was little that anyone could do to stop the arrival of H1N1. And rather than the tentative foray across the Tex-Mex line being a signature border infringement justifying the right-wing media's jeremiad, it might have been the way H1N1 ended up jumping two oceans – hopping from Veracruz to Auckland, New Zealand – that was most provocative.

In New Zealand, where I live and am writing these pages, this story captured our imagination in slightly different ways. The virus piggy-backed on the rucksacks of a group of students on a field trip in Mexico. At the end of April 2009, 25 Rangitoto College students from Auckland returned from an Easter tour of Mexico feeling ill by the time they arrived home. Eleven tested positive for influenza A, and they were immediately quarantined.[20] What made this story different from the US one was that, for once, New Zealand's situation was more broadly relevant. In an isolated, faraway country with the Lord of the Rings, milk powder, and Flight of the Conchords as the most recognizable forms of international impact, the New Zealand media is constantly trying to find angles to link world stories with its own. "New Zealand added to Google Swine Flu Map" heralded the *NZ Business Review*.[21] That the flu added to New Zealand's international prestige, in the minds of New Zealanders' minds at least, was reminiscent of Tom Lehrer's comic song "Who's Next?"[22]

There were 97 laboratory-confirmed cases of influenza A in New Zealand shortly after the students' return, and in early May, more than 300 laboratory-confirmed cases of the disease were identified worldwide.[23] The border jumping was not just national, it was also seasonal. By popping down to the antipodes, the virus avoided the northern hemisphere's warm season, which might otherwise have been its demise.

Protecting national borders might be a laudable attempt to safeguard the citizens of that nation, and in small island nations it might almost seem possible, but no nation seriously considered closing down its airports. The result of viral protectionism might be economic disaster, and according to the WHO, it would also be an infringement upon civil liberties.[24]

The idea of nation helps decide what names a particular flu epidemic should be given but also tells stories that are not quite accurate. The

1918 "Spanish" flu is a particularly good example. The deadliest of any recorded influenza epidemic, it was called "The Spanish Lady" and was widely presumed at the time to have started in Spain. However, this origin myth, came, wrote Trilla and his colleagues, as a result of the greater freedom of press present in Spain, as a neutral country during World War I.[25] While Spanish newspapers were reporting the arrival of the disease: "The US and European press, likely for political reasons, did not acknowledge or transmit timely and accurate news about the high number of casualties among their military and civilian population that were attributable to the ongoing influenza epidemic."[26] Contemporary virologists and epidemiologists, it should be said, are convinced that Spain was not the birthplace of this particular epidemic. Today, the WHO recommends that geographic locations (along with animal names, people names, and alarming adjectives) be avoided in the naming of new infectious diseases.[27]

These narratives about influenza were all about its elusive nature and how it changes shape, jumps between species, shimmies over national borders, crosses seasons, and runs back and forth between the agrarian hinterlands and the urban sprawl, out of control. Of course – and this can't be ignored – influenza also can make people very, very ill. Public health in general, and medicine in particular, told other stories to try to contain the complicated realities of influenza, but curiously, these stories were all told much more serenely. The anticipation and anxiety woven through the thriller narratives was discarded in favour of banality. The flu (not "influenza") was likely a well-worn pair of slippers, but unfortunately, slippers with unfinished seams blistering and abrading. Yes, we know which pair we have on – we've worn these before – they just don't feel good.

To start with, during the 2009 H1N1 pandemic, public health officials around the globe exhorted us to stay away from the doctor if we had "the flu." Please keep your germs at home! Self-diagnosis, as we will see in chapter 2, is not commonly part of mainstream disease awareness campaigns. Many public health initiatives focus on identifying symptom patterns that are associated with particular diseases and advising presentation to a doctor for confirmation. We've never seen, for example, posters on the bus saying: "If you have respiratory syncytial virus, stay at home!" On the other hand, we see plenty of "If you have the flu, stay at home!" This form of messaging is based on the premise that we have a shared understanding of what influenza looks like. You can probably tell from the introductory paragraphs to this chapter that there are many different ways of understanding, and telling tales about influenza in the popular mind.

In fact, this discourse (we all know what we are talking about!) has led to dramatic shifts in the diagnostic process. We are all so familiar with influenza that public health officials reassigned the roles of the various characters in the wider illness narrative. They shifted diagnostic responsibility from doctor to patient. Laypeople have been actively encouraged to diagnose themselves (see figure 1.1), and this has resulted in many more new ways to tell the story of flu.

How peculiar a tale is this, one that turns diagnosis on its head! Being sick and going to the doctor is the role of the patient. Having medical knowledge, authority, and access to health bureaucracy is the role of the doctor.[28] The doctor's professional status gives him or her permission to name disease, which once named, can be explained, treated, and hopefully cured. Usually, the power to diagnose is specifically attached to the doctor. One can't have sick leave without a doctor's note; access to antibiotics is contingent upon a medical diagnosis; insurance reimbursement and other entitlements are linked to a professional diagnosis. There is great power contained in the ability to diagnose, and "the profession which is custodian of the [diagnostic] label is ascendant."[29] To name what ails us is to have an elite sense of how the world works.

Interestingly, the medical literature on self-diagnosis of most diseases is dismissive. The lay public is seen as vulnerable, not only to quacks and charlatans but to exploitation by the pharmaceutical industry, which is keen to promote its remedies to a wider clientele and to propose and claim diagnostic labels.[30] This literature also tests lay aptitude to self-diagnose. Medicine acknowledges that in many cases self-diagnosis would be desirable if it were efficacious – in the case of malaria, for example, or altitude sickness. Treatment and prognosis would be much improved if laypeople could get a head start and confirm the diagnosis *de bonne heure*. Alas, people aren't very good at self-testing yet.

The self-diagnosis of influenza was never tested before it was promoted. It just made good sense. People know if they have the flu, don't they? A research group of which I was a member surveyed 1147 New Zealanders and found that despite having the symptoms identified by the Ministry of Health and the WHO as being suggestive of influenza, less than a quarter of those who had self-diagnosed the flu actually had

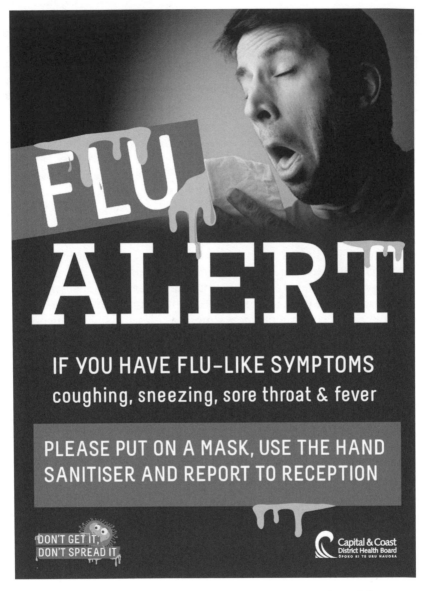

1.1 Public health warnings presume a familiarity with, and the reliability of, influenza case definition criteria. [Used with permission of Capital & Coast District Health Board – photo credit: Flickr/foshydog]

serological evidence of influenza infection.[31] Here, influenza has once again redrawn boundaries: the layperson has been invited, against usual medical practices, to take on the authoritative role of diagnostician. But this intrusion is not told as a tale of suspense. Rather it is paradoxical, on the basis of the taken-for-granted lay understanding of the diagnosis.

The story of influenza as recounted above is one of shape-shifting and boundary crossing, in the material nature of the virus, in its disdain for social boundaries, and in the human response to its presence. It underlines the slippery nature of this physical diagnosis, and the complexities it entails. In the popular imagination, however, influenza has a strangely firm foundation. *Flu* is a word we all know, a disease we can all recognize, an illness for which we have explanations, descriptions, and treatments. To say one is "feeling fluey" as one might say in the Commonwealth, or to have a "mild flu" as one might say in the United States, is to make a clear assertion of well-boundaried symptoms: shivery and weak, worse than a cold, risky, but probably OK. Most of us don't know anyone who has died of the flu, even though we have heard about the ravages of the 1918 flu epidemic and are regularly reminded of its deadly potential by the media. Flu exists in forms that have little to do with the morphology or symptomatology of the influenza virus infection.

While I was writing this chapter, numerous interested friends shared their explanations and formulae for distinguishing flu from cold. "You know it's the flu when you don't care whether you live or die"; "you know it's the flu when you have those bad muscle aches"; or "you just *know* when you have the flu!"

As Philip Hugh-Jones wrote in 1973: "In Britain patients will often say that they 'had a touch of the 'flu,' just as in the tropics they will say they had malaria, simply meaning, in either case, that they felt ill and presumed they had a fever. So, it is interesting to know what true influenza is really like."[32] But while medicine still hasn't figured this out, laypeople have. Lindsey Prior and his team have written about lay certainty surrounding flu. In their study of 54 older people describing the difference between the flu and a cold, they found that flu was associated with behavioural correlates.[33] What you were or were not able to do indicated whether you had the flu or a cold. If you couldn't get out of bed, or go to work, it was the flu. His participants described symptoms that were not generally considered part of the medical description of the disease and described colds as being potential stepping stones to influenza. But importantly, flu was a "whole of the body" illness, rather than something confined to the head, like a cold.

There isn't much doubt, in lay terms, about what the flu is. It's recognizable enough that it is included in fiction, without the author needing to explain it. It is readily recognized from a brief sketch of symptoms. In Hemingway's "A Day's Wait," the young boy has the flu. He "was shivering, his face was white, and he walked slowly as though it ached to move."[34] Similarly, Richard Leibmann-Smith was able to satirize influenza in this 1976 *New Yorker* piece on the basis of general familiarity with its symptoms, paired with recognition of its pathogenesis: "Swine Flu is a disease that people can relate to. Headache, nausea, fever – nothing too deep, symptomwise. It's not trying to be the new Yellow Fever."[35]

The terms "flu" and "influenza-type illness" are widely used to replace influenza itself. They are, in effect, condensed images, or simplified stories, that stand for the complex materiality of viral infection and its pathophysiological consequences. Laypersons, like medics, are inclined to want to think of flu as being "influenza-like" because recognition is so important to its control. It would be so much better if influenza could be "just so." But it isn't.

In the survey of self-diagnosis I mentioned on the previous page, we matched a list of symptoms to those participants who had accurately self-diagnosed their influenza; only the runny nose and fatigue correlated with positive self-diagnosis. Not very helpful for public health officials!

Even in our study of self-diagnosis, people were very good at recognizing what influenza was *supposed* to be like. Those who met the case definitions of influenza-like illness were much more likely to believe they had influenza, even though they didn't.

Doctors aren't averse to talking about flu either. Close to three thousand articles in the PubMed database have the word *flu* in their titles, making reference to influenza. Hence the word has an interesting rhetorical status. Not quite a sobriquet (even though it is a shortened form of the word *influenza*, it's not the same thing) nor a metaphor (it is too close to influenza to be different enough from it), *flu* nonetheless plays an important role in communicating and in shaping how both patients and doctors feel about disease.

Michael Hanne has written that "while medical professionals in the West willingly accept that stories and metaphors play a large part in the thinking of laypeople, and consequently in communications between themselves and their patients, there is some reluctance to acknowledge that biomedical science itself is largely organized in narrative and, especially, metaphorical terms."[36] He also notes: "It is highly desirable for metaphorical models and narrative scenarios to be developed and employed in the mass media that will improve the validity of folk wisdom, have a positive effect on people's understanding and behavior before they get sick, and allow them to bring with them better mental models whenever they come to a doctor with health concerns."[37]

These oppositional narrative genres relating to influenza have a socially understandable foundation (but often challenging social consequences). To contain influenza, or any other infectious agent, one of the first important steps is being able to count cases. National surveillance programs around the world keep tallies of the number of people stricken by the disease. We count those who present to their doctor with influenza-like symptoms, as well as those who, more gravely ill, find their way into our hospital beds. The count takes place via diagnosis. How many cases of *this* as opposed to *that*. The figures thus collected are reported back to our various ministries and departments of health, who in turn feed this information to the WHO.

Influenza monitoring starts with an idea of what influenza should be: the defining of joints to which Arnold referred.[38] A doctor is unlikely to write in his or her notes "patient suffering from influenza." The convention is to refer to "influenza-like illness." This phrase has a standard (agreed-upon) meaning: the patient presents with a temperature of 100°F (37.8°C) or more, and a cough or a sore throat, in the absence of a known cause other than influenza.[39] Yet 30% of influenza infections will be symptom-free – not influenza-like at all.[40] In addition, comparison of influenza symptoms across nations reveals that the same influenza virus feels to different people in different places.[41] In a Moroccan sample, 16% suffered from nausea, in China, 1.9%. Abnormalities on chest radiography were more common in the Moroccan cohort than in either the United States or China (26.3% versus 5.1% in China and 7.1% in the United States).[42] And finally, interviews with confirmed influenza sufferers of similar demographic and from the same community revealed no particular symptom patterns, no dominant symptoms, and widely varying degrees of severity.[43]

So "influenza-like illness" isn't necessarily influenza. It's just the closest we normally get to pinning this virus down in the outpatient setting. In hospital, however, where the patient is likely to be extremely unwell, we're far more likely to go to the lab to confirm our suspicion that a patient is suffering from influenza: diagnosis plays an important role in identifying the appropriate treatment. Hence, in principle, hospitals should have accurate records of influenza infection. And, in the hospital, staff can record these positive diagnoses, finally getting a firm head count. But hospital coding is yet another location where medicine's attempts to contain include incongruous disregard for classificatory boundaries.

The clinical coding department is where the count takes place. Clinical coders apply guidelines issued by the WHO and subsequently interpreted by each nation's ministry of health. Coders peruse medical notes and either record the code chosen by the clinician or select an appropriate code from the information supplied. The codes applied come from the ICD, currently in its 11th revision (ICD-11). But given the quickly mutating nature of influenza, there isn't necessarily a code ready for each new configuration. Sometimes an old one must do.

In the 2005 avian influenza pandemic, coders used the code J-09: "Influenza due to identified avian influenza virus." However, since no one died from it, little use was made of that code by coding departments. Faced with the 2009 H1N1 pandemic, the ICD Update and Reference Committee decided that there was no need to create a new code. Coders were instructed to use the hitherto underused 2005 code, J-09 (avian virus), to record any deaths by H1N1 ("swine flu"). The Committee recognized the irony of letting pigs fly, requiring coders to make the free text entry: "Influenza A H1N1 – confirmed."[44] They also made a nod towards Ockham, recognizing that they had been hasty when they had established J-09 in 2005. It would have been wiser to have been less specific, in order to give space for emerging influenza strains. Reflecting this reality, the code has since been altered, and no longer refers to "Influenza due to identified *avian* influenza," but to "*certain* identified influenza virus."

This classificatory challenge is not completely surprising. Mildred Blaxter described the ICD as history, "a museum of past and present concepts of the nature of disease."[45] It's a complicated matter, trying to develop a classificatory scheme for the medicine: "No activity so complex as medicine, however or with so long a history, can achieve so logical a conclusion: throughout the ages the system has proceeded from the parts to the whole, building layer upon successive layer and reorganizing only partially and intermittently."[46]

Even though H1N1 is now anchored in a sensible code, it hasn't kept its name. As one might have expected, it has shifted shape once again. Even though its morphology has not changed, its status has, and it is now defined not as a pandemic influenza, but as a seasonal one. The WHO has afforded it a new nomenclature: A(H1N1)pdm09.[47] We continue to catch the flu, and it's always the same one, but at the same time, it's quite a different story.

We still need to be able to shape the story of influenza, despite its amorphous nature. Finding a way to speak about it effectively is important to the improvement of health outcomes and requires a range of voices. Returning to history for a moment, Michael Bresalier, in his accounting of the early microbial history of influenza, described the diagnostic definition of influenza as one where different forms of knowledge were aligned. Various arms of British medicine (epidemiological, clinical, public health) saw influenza with different perspectives and different tools. However, "each provided the other with conceptual and practical resources, and with specific problems to solve."[48]

We have a range of different storytellers and resources that shape the diagnosis as we know it. What is simultaneously curious and helpful is that the metaphors and metonyms of influenza and the ways in which we talk about it involve so many different ways of knowing: those of the virologist, the epidemiologist, the general practitioner, the media, and (more than is probably acknowledged) the layperson. That there are so many ways to tell the flu story matters. It matters because we need to be alert to the story's authorship and its intended audience. Calling it *flu* provides one form of capture and in some cases a useful one.

However, in other cases, it is not so useful. During the H1N1 pandemic, there were reports of deaths and serious morbidity from other illnesses linked to the incorrect presumption of influenza infection.[49] The death of Zachary Gravatt in New Zealand is a case in point. This young medical student died from meningococcal meningitis, identified initially as a bad case of the flu. He was sent by his doctor to the hospital with what the coroner reported as "flu-like symptoms" and died that evening. The coroner explained that the doctor on service "could not find an obvious explanation to the symptoms and considered the H1N1 flu as the most likely cause, given Zachary's exposure to the virus."[50] The presumption of influenza was maintained even in the presence of a negative influenza test, and the patient's worsening condition: the guiding narrative of influenza-like illness during a pandemic was simply too strong to allow for other potential explanations. The coroner's post-mortem recommendations included that in the future front-line staff should also consider bacterial sepsis (meningococcal disease) in the presence of influenza-like illness.

Flu allows us to capture the elusive influenza virus, but it can also, as it did with the young New Zealander, release from contemplation other stories of other diseases that have clearer identities and unequivocal consequences. Medical educators have yet another metaphor for describing this unleashing. It's called *anchoring*. When a patient presents with a particular set of symptoms, the clinician may anchor the diagnostic hypothesis in an initial assessment. The metaphorical anchor signifies the pursuit by the diagnostician of the safe haven of certainty. Once the clinician identifies a pattern, he or she seeks to confirm the diagnosis, "selectively marshalling" information to support the presumed condition, and subconsciously rejecting subtle indicators of other diagnostic possibilities.[51]

Returning to my departure point, flu exercises its powerful organizing influence precisely because it is so common. It is an example of a diagnosis we all understand. Just saying "I've got the flu" makes so much sense that little more need be said. It's the shorthand that I referred to in the Introduction which, with just one (part of) a word speaks volumes. "I've got the flu" means something like "I've got something that makes me feel pretty sick all over, which is probably contagious, and that I should normally recover from." But it is nowhere near as tidy as having a name suggests it would be and in this way provides a wonderful example of the limitations of diagnosis as a way of approaching disease.

We could unpack any one of the diagnostic labels that we wouldn't want to receive – the kind of diagnoses that when said out loud, or announced to someone we care about, makes us cringe – in the same way as I just have influenza. Cancer, for example. It has its own nickname – "the Big C" – and it's as elusive as the flu. Cancer is not one disease even though we talk about it as if it were. It is a collection of many diseases, in many different locations with many different prognoses. Even breast cancer, which sounds like one disease, is made up of all sorts of different kinds of abnormal cellular activity, in all different parts of the breast. The word *cancer* by itself means far less from a medical perspective than it means from a social, a cultural, or an emotional one. The diagnosis of cancer includes conditions ranging from simple, treatable, and limited afflictions, to chronic, long-term disorders requiring ongoing care, but also, and importantly, to diseases that are most likely to be fatal in the very short term. And even within the subcategory of likely-to-be-fatal-in-the-very-short-term, there is unexpected variation and resistance.[52]

The metaphors used to discuss cancer are different than those of influenza, but are just as powerful. While we "catch" the flu, we "battle" cancer. With cancer, we become survivors, previvors. With flu, we "get over it."

Less than a century ago, it would have been a different disease that would have provoked the anxiety and the kinds of storytelling that the cancer diagnosis now elicits. The uncertainty associated with cancer today (How long will I live? Will this treatment save me or kill me?) is similar to what was previously associated with the failing heart or the labile blood sugar. In 1942, Dr Sachs wrote: "I have long since stopped predicting death as inevitable in the presence of heart disease … I refuse to alarm the patient and have him or her know whether the pressure is five or ten points higher or lower. The doctor should know; the patient need not know."[53]

Cancer provides a particularly good example of how a diagnosis can be imbued with transformative power. However, it is not more serious than a range of other ailments. In a paper about diagnostic disclosure protocols, F. Bettevy, herself a cancer patient, editorializes: "Today, a cancer diagnosis is no longer a death warrant. Patients want to be able to believe in a medical reality that carries the hope of long remission and even cure."[54]

Diagnosis always occupies an important place in the story of an illness. It frequently marks the end of one metaphorical chapter and the start of a new one, largely because of its presumed link to prognosis. Returning to the words of Hippocrates (in the Introduction), the diagnosis was a window to the prognosis, the expectation for the future. And this access to a putative certainty was what gave medicine (doctors) their power. But the certainty of diagnosis does not necessarily predict the outcome of the disease with the same certainty. Charles Lund underlined in his highly cited 1946 paper titled "The Doctor, the Patient and the Truth" that upon announcing a diagnosis, the doctor still does "not know at this time and has no further tests to differentiate the potentially cured patients from the potential failures."[55] It is too difficult to really know what will happen, he writes. This uncertainty is fundamental in structuring both power relations and the impact of diagnosis.

Antonella Surbone, both philosopher and oncologist muses: "Stressing certainty over uncertainty in prognostication betrays the complexity of life. It seems that we are again trying to reify disease, and to distance all subjective elements from the doctor-patient relationship."[56] As ontological as may appear the diagnosis, as tight as may seem its link to treatment and to the future, diagnoses are funny things with porous boundaries.[57] Our desire to palliate uncertainty via diagnosis may lead to, rather than remedy, its powerful impact.

The elusive nature of diagnosis does not dilute the vigour with which individuals will pursue diagnostic explanations for their disorders. Chapter 2 describes how a diagnosis starts in a patient story and is exchanged for a medical one. This process of narrative exchange can be fraught as a result of the different storytelling perspectives and the respective weight given each one. Medical and lay stories do not always align, nor do they result in the same denouement. Let's turn the page to discuss self-diagnosis and how it confirms particular forms of authority.

CHAPTER TWO

Whose Stories?
Narrative Exchange and Self-Diagnosis

The diagnostic process may be a moment in which separate stories are stitched together to create a neatly joined assembly, or one of contest when stories – the sick person, the doctors, and an entire panoply of external ones – collide. It may be a narrative duel that extends beyond the doctor's office to include the family, the colleagues, all narrating diagnosis in their own ways. It may equally be a moment in which stories are exchanged and elaborated, constructed, and told together. How the story is told, heard, and acknowledged has a profound impact on the experience of illness.

Any time people go to the doctor, they start telling a story even before they get there. They have to connect some dots. The discomfort they are feeling or problem they are experiencing must have, for them to seek medical advice, some relationship to what they believe the work of doctors to be.

This connecting of dots, however the individual or those around him propose to organize the problem, and the interpretive angle they've decided to take is the beginning of a story that is going to be taken to the doctor. When the doctor turns to the individuals and says, "So what brings you here today?" the patients assemble the events that made them think they should talk with a health professional and weave them together so they will make sense.[1] A sore throat can just as easily be attributed to bad cooking, heart burn, reflux, or a heart attack. And it's often this way.

For your sore hands, you tell her about your mother's, and how her hands were gnarled with osteoarthritis. You talk about the persistent discomfort in your left pointer finger, your right pinkie. You explain that you can't get your wedding ring off any more, because your joints are swollen. As you put these bits together, and explain the events, you offer the doctor the building blocks out of which the diagnostic narrative will emerge.

Of course, you could tell a different story for the same set of events and problems, and it need not be about diagnosis. There are other ways of framing hand pain. Even though your mother's hands were gnarled with osteoarthritis, you only started noticing your hand pain when you got your new mountain bike. You love your new bike, and you're now biking every day. You have been trying to take more risks, so you're gripping your break levers ferociously. Your wedding ring is misshapen from the levers. The brake system was slightly different from the one on your old bike. You return to your bike mechanic and ask him to replace the brakes with what you had before. You think that will work better for your grip.

Just as easily, one can attribute a gastric upset to someone's cooking rather than to a potential disease; a headache to stress; a sore joint to poor fitness; even, maybe slightly unreasonably, a fever to overwork. But when a problem goes to the doctor, chances are the individual has made a decision that there's a diagnosis to be had, and the story is already starting to take a particular frame. However, this particular process of storytelling is the first step in initiating a transformation, of empowering diagnosis. By seeking the diagnostic explanation, its linkages and explanations, we are voluntarily disrupting our own stories. We have to give them away, expose them, and listen to their not-necessarily-to-our-liking retelling to get a diagnosis.

But this moment of exchange is not as simple as "the individual tells/ the doctor retells." Not everyone is a good storyteller, and not every patient knows the conventions of diagnostic narrative. They may, for example, expect the body to be able to provide more information than language and leave the clinician to construct a story without enough help. They may not have precision in their vocabulary to explain how they feel, or the nature/intensity of their pain. They may resort to standardized scales: "It was bad. It was an 8!" or "I don't know. It was just, well, sore …" without being able to describe, contextualize, or link. When a patient can't tell the story, can't express concerns effectively, the doctor-listener may need to coax the story along, wrangling it up and herding it, hoping all the while, he or she has the right elements gathered up in the right paddock.

But in the ideal rendition of this narrative exchange, the story one brings to the doctor for diagnostic purposes is heard (hopefully), processed, rearranged, and retold. Balint, in his classical text on the doctor-patient interaction describes this exchange as a "negotiation," where patient and doctor reflect upon the telling and retelling and together shape the new story until it takes a form that both can live with.[2] It's a cooperative undertaking. Leder, on the other hand, describes the diagnostic process as an "interpretive" endeavour, in which the diagnostician takes the narrative and completes it with technological, experiential, and physical texts to develop a diagnostic explanation.[3] He cautions medicine against losing the patient narrative – the representation of illness – from sight.

When Frank writes about the offering of a narrative by the person seeking medical care, he calls it a "narrative surrender." It is the point, he writes, at which medicine wrests control from the individual and transforms a story of dysfunction into a medical one. The language changes, the explanatory framework shifts, and diagnosis replaces the symptoms in the framing of the illness.[4]

Frank, Leder, and many others have pointed to the transfer of the patient's narrative, the "taking" of the patient history, as salient and problematic. As Frank explains, "more is involved in [the illness experience] than the medical story can tell,"[5] and he argues that for most people, there is a need to go beyond the medical narrative to recover their own voice.[6] Fear of having their narrative usurped by the medicalized version may push patients to try to control the diagnostic process. They may not want to relinquish their stories, or they may relinquish them but so completely formed as to resist interference by their physicians.

The medical profession remains the primary go-to point for diagnosis, but its dominant authority in this regard has shown some cracks. Doctors are no longer the only professionals who have sole authority to diagnose. A range of other professions, including the chiropractor, nurse practitioner, or physiotherapist, may diagnose certain conditions in some countries. Furthermore, the nature of the relationship between doctors and patients sees patients more willing to challenge their doctor, dispute findings, or seek advice outside of the doctor-patient relationship.[7]

But it is not just the changing status of medicine that leads laypeople to more vigorously engage themselves in the diagnostic process.

Pharmaceutical companies also present compelling stories about diagnoses to the public, hoping to encourage them to see themselves as characters in the proposed stories. If they do so, they will in turn present a narrative to their doctor that may direct his or her thinking towards the diagnosis for which the pharmaceutical company is marketing the cure. It's also a terrific workaround for those companies working in countries who do not permit direct-to-consumer advertising. They can advertise the remedy directly to the physicians – that's authorized – and instead, just promote disease awareness through the identifiable stories.

One powerful example of this commercial storytelling focuses on female sexuality. The pharmaceutical industry has been very actively looking for the "pink Viagra," that is to say, a medication, targeting women, that would have the same commercial success as has sildenafil (marketed as Viagra).[8] To locate and develop interest in a female condition equivalent to erectile dysfunction, a number of industry players focused on something called *hypoactive sexual desire disorder* in which the person thus diagnosed asserts low libido which interferes with her social well-being. Rather than advertise the medication itself however, its patent owners created marketing vignettes, telling the stories of women who "came out" as suffering from low sexual drive and relating its symptoms. The idea was to encourage viewers to see themselves in these stories and, in turn, recount them to their doctors.[9]

Figures 2.1 and 2.2 provide examples of the long-standing history of pharmaceutical industry storytelling. Both are self-explanatory, because they use powerful visual storytelling tools. The historical advertisement for *Fer Bravais*, an iron supplement, focuses on the plight of the woman suffering from anemia (*anémie*). She is weary and exhausted and cannot fulfil her social role. The image is designed to draw the consumer in to a similar story, projecting herself in the role of the exhausted seamstress. The contemporary advertisement is not for a substance per se. As is common in contemporary pharmaceutical industry marketing, the object of the advertisement is not the medication itself but awareness of the condition. In this case, the product this advertisement intends to promote is not yet approved for non-experimental use, but its promoters probably believe that the approval and public release is not far away. The first step in the promotion of the medication is to focus on the disorder for which it intends to provide a remedy.

The image shown in figure 2.2 tells the story of the powerful subject constrained by chronic migraine. This image is one of liberation and of empowerment. It directs its readers to a webpage produced by Allergan

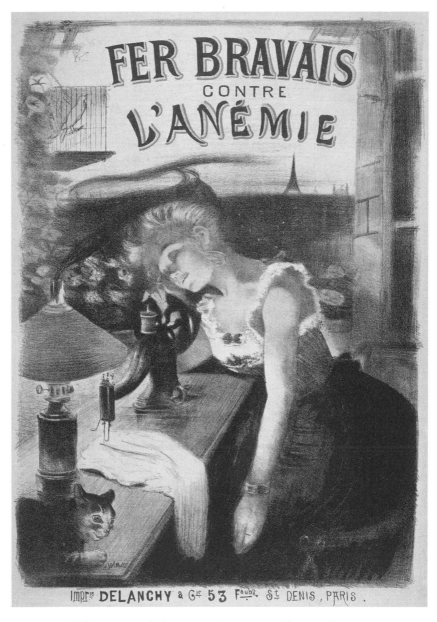

2.1 Selling a remedy by promoting a story: The visual narrative
of the weary woman, unable to fulfil her social role. [Adolphe-Léon Willette,
ca. 1890. Credit: Wellcome Collection]

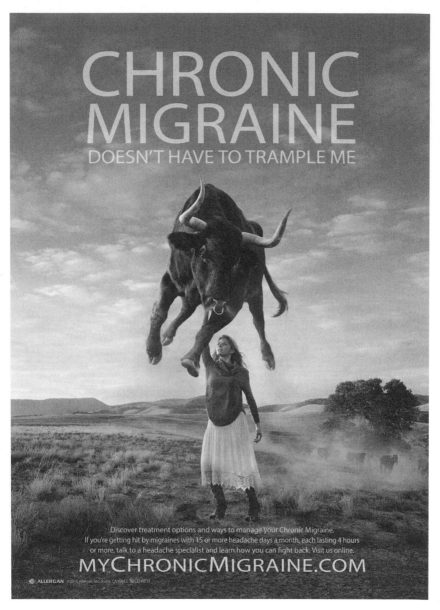

2.2 A contemporary marketing narrative: The empowered woman behind the migraine. [Credit: © Allergen. Used with permission. All rights reserved.]

(at the time I draft these words, currently working on the development of a medication targeting the calcitonin gene-related peptide – a new approach to the bedevilling problem of migraine), which at the same time invites viewers to think of their personal narrative in these terms of empowerment, and it provides self-diagnosis and self-management tools.

However, possibly the most important factor in the act of self-diagnosis is the social importance of the diagnosis in making sense of health, disease, and illness. More and more perhaps (but also previously), as Balint wrote in the 1960s, "*The request for a name for the illness, for a diagnosis* is the most pressing problem for the patient. It is only in the second instance that the patient asks for therapy ... finding 'nothing wrong' is no answer to the patient's most burning demand for a demand for a name for his illness."[10] The power to name is, according to sociologist Phil Brown, core to social control.[11] Self-diagnosis narratives are thus central to an individual's need to anchor the explanation of dysfunction in acceptable medical terms and to maintain control.

But stories anchored in self-diagnosis mess with the traditional, medically mediated narrative order. In the traditional story, patients present symptoms (events) for interpretation by the doctor. In the self-diagnosis story, however, patients make links and identify associations without involving the doctor until the very last minute (when they have no choice, if they require the sick leave, the prescription, the insurance reimbursement). The story of self-diagnosis is one both of resistance – if not of defiance! – as it proposes a ready-made explanation rather than requesting a bespoke one.

Look at the "Dr Google" phenomenon, for example. The term *Dr Google* started appearing in the early years of the twenty-first century and has since become effective short hand (a story in itself) to signify the idea that patients have made up their mind about what ails them in the Internet environment rather than in the doctor's office. Lisa Gualtieri described it as transforming the *doctor* into the "second opinion" with the Internet serving as the first.[12]

In the eyes of medicine, this reversal of the narrative order is an affront to professional authority, a cause of great concern for doctors. While the patients are connecting the dots in relation to what ails them, doctors are connecting another set of dots. Explaining the threat to their diagnostic role, and the unfamiliar presence of the patient in their designated space, they tell stories about self-diagnosis and its risks. These stories hinge on the vulnerability of the layperson and the potential for their exploitation by devious non-doctors and the pharmaceutical industry. Doctors cast the non-doctors as scheming profit mongers who have proposed an alternative reason to visit the doctor: not to request a diagnosis, but to demand treatment for the condition from which, they are already convinced, they suffer.

And, of course, it's not as simple as what I've just described. There are potential harms to people and to the system when unethical, unsubstantiated or misunderstood claims shape the stories that patients may tell about what ails them. Doctors have a social brief, as well as a clinical one. As guardians of medicine, we like to see them, as they see themselves, ever vigilant against misappropriations of medical information, malicious incursions into the health system or exploitation of the ailing individual: a challenge and not an easy one!

So, it can be a bit of a narrative duel, when the stakes are set as they are. On the one hand, the doctor is the guarantor of medical authority; on the other, patients need agency to control their story. The stakes for both are difficult to reconcile. In this chapter, we look specifically at how the medical professionals report this duel. We will see what stories doctors tell us about the stories that patients tell them. These medical accounts create a kind of metanarrative about the locus of authority and what the diagnostic moment should look like. They also create an inspiring picture of what a doctor should look like. The diagnostician does not necessarily see him or herself as the agent of power and authority, as might the self-diagnosee, but rather as a vigilant and caring clinician burdened by the heavy weight of diagnostic responsibility.

These medical stories about patients' self-diagnoses are not the new genre we might have suspected. While contemporary doctors are very vocal about the Dr Google effect, their predecessors were concerned about the same phenomenon, albeit via different media. The very personification (complete with professional title) of what is in fact an impersonal Internet interaction demonstrates the degree to which contemporary medicine sees self-diagnosis as a threat or a foe with a living, breathing impact on the layperson. While the personification is new, doctor comments about patient incursion into the diagnostic process are not. As early as the late nineteenth century, doctors fretted about patients trying to figure out what ailed them on their own. Just like contemporary physicians, they argued that the patient who was influenced by information from outside the doctor's office was generally made very anxious. Not only this, their proposed diagnoses put at risk the very work of the doctor and his or her ability to think clearly. The plot of the self-diagnosis narrative is based in Agon, a contest between not the doctor and the patient, rather between the doctor and the evil forces seeking to conquer the poor patient via external diagnosis.

The idea that free-circulating information about serious medical conditions would upset the layperson surfaced in the early twentieth century, if not before. For example, in 1934, the surgeon, Albert Krecke wrote "[the patient] has heard so much about all manner of diseases that every time he feels a little poorly, he imagines the worst." He noted that not all preoccupations were problematic: "It is comparatively harmless that he should fear inflammation of the lungs as soon as he feels a slight shooting pain the chest, and appendicitis whenever he has a stomach-ache … But those who come to the doctor because they think they may have cancer are the most tormented of all. A harmless soreness on the tongue, a slight smart in the mammary gland, an innocent haemorrhoidal nodule, are attributed to cancer."[13] The assault on the worried well might come from newspapers, editorialized one author in the *British Medical Journal* (now *BMJ*), writing that they would "alarm a reader with slight digestive symptoms by suggesting to him that the dreaded acid has already begun its deadly work."[14]

However, beyond the fact that patients tended to become anxious as a result of their readings or discussions outside of the doctors' rooms, the doctors themselves were encouraged to be very careful about how they received information from these anxious patients. Their self-diagnostic pronouncements could sway even the best trained doctors of today. Robert Gersuny, also a surgeon, reminded both patient and doctor that what the patient says "is not an objective exposition of the case, but the opinion he himself has formed regarding his own condition, and this opinion should not be allowed to influence the doctor's judgement."[15] Dr Robert Keith, in his 1918 manual on "case-taking" echoed this, pointing out that "a patient may give a diagnosis of his own, but you must never accept this without making full examination; on the other hand, you should listen patiently to what he has to say; you should ever be kind and sympathetic if you wish to gain and retain a patient's confidence."[16] He pointed out that patients could be "long-winded and irrelevant, and too much time should not be spent on this point."[17]

Pushing this point at newly graduated physicians, Dr R. Lapham maintained that patients who thought they knew what was wrong with them were a challenge to doctors and could lead the doctor down false trails and garden paths: "The history which is begun by the patient giving his own diagnosis is very apt to be a hindrance rather than a help to the physician, and when a history is so begun the physician must ever be on his guard lest he unconsciously follow along the line of reasoning of the patient, or allow himself to be prejudiced or influenced by the diagnosis given by the patient. Well should we know that pathology which the patient may describe by saying, 'I'm having indigestion,' or, 'I'm having trouble with my stomach,' may not even lie below the diaphragm. Accepting such a statement from a patient may very well mean that the physician begins by following the trail of completely false or non-existent pathology."[18]

Doctors also related the degree to which the patients' preconceived ideas about what ailed them interfered with the doctor-patient relationship as well as what doctors believed their own work should be. Gersuny was rather blunt in his assertion that "sick people who imagine that they know the exact nature of their ailment, or who have read up their complaint in some book, are a great source of trouble to their doctors and themselves. The practitioner must find out what they think their malady is and try to prove to them that their conclusions are incorrect, and to make it clear that they must cease from analysing and brooding over their symptoms."[19] This assertion is an example of what I referred to above, a way of righting the keel and putting the public back on the track preferred by doctors, where the boundaries were clear, and each got on with their respective role in relation to arriving upon a diagnosis. Patients were to put themselves in the doctors' hands, and leave them free to come up with the name of the disorder.

Numerous publications sought to teach the public how to be good patients and to explain what they should expect from their doctors. Once such example, *The Public and the Doctor* by Dr Berthold Hadra, instructed patients how to be responsible. He penned: "The practicing physician cannot help wondering how little accurate and correct information the general public possesses as to medical affairs ... As a natural consequence the position and work of the physician is greatly encumbered, and a sound relationship between the public and him endangers, to the detriment and annoyance of both."[20] Another much later publication with the same aim saw it as a failure of medicine that "the patient is easily persuaded by some enthusiast in his circle of family or friends to try this or that health scheme, to consult some non-medical 'healer.'"[21]

The consequence of what these doctors believed was patient misinformation was ineffective or poorly controlled treatment. In 1878, Dr

Juke de Styrap, who is remembered for his work on the code of ethics of the British Medical Association, complained that a patient should be obedient to the instructions of his doctor and remain "uninfluenced by his own or other crude opinions, as to their fitness – for a failure in any one particular may render an otherwise judicious plan of treatment hurtful, and even dangerous."[22] Gersuny prompted doctors to make sure to disabuse patients of their misconceived ideas, because otherwise "it may happen that after a while, the patient will direct the treatment ... the doctor's influence is at an end."[23]

Also worried about the impact of lay input into treatment (some 35 years later), Dr William Bainbridge of New York expressed concerns in relation to cancer treatment. He felt that the public should be safeguarded from medical debates because of the false hope premature assertions about this or that therapy could instil. He wrote: "If a lay man reads, for example, or hears that 'while radium *manifestly* (the italics are mine[24]) *ought to replace surgery in many instances*' ... he is fairly sure to conclude that the author of such a statement means that radium can and does cure at least some cases which surgery is powerless to benefit. Yet how many such cases can be presented? Are we fighting cancer with *facts* when we make such assertions, even among ourselves?"[25]

Many of the writers assigned responsibility for lay misuse of medical information to profit seekers: "The newspaper press, so powerful in the correction of many crying abuses, is unfortunately too ready for the sake of lucre to aid and abet the enormities of quackery by the insertion of its offensive advertisements," explained de Styrap. "Medical men, individually and collectively would direct the special attention of the editors and proprietors of newspapers, and of periodicals in general, to the immoral tendency and contaminating effect produced upon the youth and purity of the country by the disgusting 'quack' pamphlets which are advertised and disseminated far and wide through the medium of the press," he continued. He further insisted that patients "should never allow themselves to be persuaded to take medicines recommended to them by the self-constituted doctors and doctoresses so frequently met with in society, and who assume to possess infallible remedies for the cure of this or that disease."[26]

The belief in what an unidentified author in the *British Medical Journal* referred to as "commerce without conscience" persisted well into the next century. Self-diagnosis and self-medication were "encouraged by advertisements of proprietary medicines in the popular press. These habits, in addition to causing in many cases a very unfortunate or even fatal delay in summoning skilled medical assistance, often result in direct physical injury of a serious kind."[27] Or, as a Dr Brown warned in 1862: "Neither can the Quack give you his kingdoms of health, even though you worship him as he best likes, by paying him for his trash; he is dangerous and dear, and often deadly, – have nothing to do with him."[28]

The matter of "non-scientifically trained" health care providers alarmed doctors writing about self-diagnosis and lay incursions into the preserve of medical information. Indeed, the American Medical Association was established in 1846 in response to growing worries about quackery and unfounded health claims by "unqualified practitioners." Diagnostic skill was what differentiated the doctor from the quack, proclaimed Dr E.G. Little in his lecture at St George's Medical School: "The fatal weakness of the unqualified practitioner is not his lack of a medical degree, but his lack of knowledge of disease which, however imperfectly, enables a qualified man to interpret the signs presented by this patient, to distinguish one sign from another, and to relate the signs to prognosis and treatment."[29]

The absence of adequate patient knowledge and understanding of anatomy and pathology opened the gate to the potential for quackery, wrote Sir Henry Brackenbury, vice president of the British Medical Association, explaining that it was "no trivial matter; for it is not only a serious obstacle to a doctor giving a rational explanation or description to a patient of his condition – so often and so naturally demanded – but is the major cause of all the superstition, quackery, charlatanism, and nonsense in reference to medical matters still so astonishingly prevalent among persons who, in other spheres of which they have more knowledge are able to think logically and well."[30]

Contemporary doctors renew these same masterplots. Rather than speak of "commerce without conscience," they discuss the "Dr Google phenomenon." In place of quacks, they are concerned about alternative therapists. They describe self-diagnosis as an obstacle for the diligent physician to overcome, a trap into which patient and doctor can fall. It sets the physician up to misdiagnosis, disrupts the patient-doctor relationship,[31] and increases anxiety.[32] It is underpinned by the exploitative actions of industry such as big pharma, big data, and big food) and more.[33] They even resort to their favourite tool – diagnosis – to discuss this debate, coining the term *cyberchondria* to refer to health anxiety generated, or augmented by, Internet use for health information.

Even though access to medical information by laypeople is not a new phenomenon, it has assumed a new persona, one that feels more pervasive, invasive, and disordering to contemporary health care providers. There are web, apps, and direct-to-consumer advertising, which replace concern about newspaper press's "pursuit of lucre," the patent drug advertisements, and "enormities of Quackery" of the last centuries.[34]

The stories doctors tell today about self-diagnosis are, for the most part, very similar to those told by doctors from the previous era. The dominant plot in these stories is of an unscrupulous for-profit industry vying for the ignorant patient's attention, scornful of the important work of medicine. Lay ignorance is variably forgiven as often as regarded with contempt, and thus, accounts of the patient behaviours waver between sympathy and impatience. There is, however, a slightly new vocabulary to describe the patients. They might be called *the worried well* afflicted with *cyberchondria* or *health anxiety disorder*. They are likely to be well-educated and have time to think about their disorders. They are still seen in the same paradoxical way by contemporary doctors as they would have been by their predecessors, as simultaneously irritants and vulnerable victims, manipulated by external forces.

Glasgow physician Des Spence characterizes these worried well as "educated patients, perhaps with too much time on their hands, who repeatedly attend the surgery with reams of Internet pages. Dr Google always diagnoses possible cancer or an appalling life-shortening degenerative condition, catastrophising all symptoms, irrespective of the probability."[35] Redolent of Krecke's historical depiction, Spence explains that the "worried well are anxious about their health, unwilling to accept reassurance, demanding investigation and referrals. They then suffer unnecessary intervention and overtreatment with real lasting harm."

His gripe is with a society that turns people into worriers. The call for useless screening, the commercial interest to sell treatments for specific conditions, and the proliferation of online information all create a perfect storm in which high-achieving patients will be compelled to see their problems in terms of diagnosis and in terms that they are determined to control.

Like his colleagues of yesteryear, Spence and numerous contemporary doctors describe an impervious foe who pushes and prods patients towards self-diagnostic conclusions, encouraging them to turn their back on well-trained physicians. These doctors protest the validity of the external information, which looks scientific enough to the unsuspecting layperson, but alas is nonsense. It's phony. It's untested. It's deceptive, they cry.

Harrison and Kouzel proclaim that "bogus information may appear in the guise of genuine evidence-based medicine and is often flanked by marketing ploys offering miraculous treatments,"[36] while Spence, again, raises his voice to say, "The truth is that these apps and devices are untested and unscientific and they will open the door of uncertainty. Make no mistake: diagnostic uncertainty ignites extreme anxiety in people. We must reflect on what we might lose here, rather than what we might gain. Will apps simply empower patients to over-diagnosis and anxiety?"[37]

Dr Tanya Feke, speaking from the Internet environment (the very soapbox she critiques), proclaims the oft-repeated axiom that non-medical information is shaping a self-diagnosis crisis that must be vanquished. Dr Google, she announces, uses outdated content and biased information. He has no experience and provides no evidence to support his claims. He should be sued for malpractice!

Dr Feke is most concerned about how online guidance of the patient interferes with the doctor-patient relationship: "It can lead to people questioning their doctor's judgment even after they have been properly seen and examined. I admit my heart plummets when I hear the words, 'but I read it on the Internet,' at the end of a visit. While I appreciate that someone wants to be proactive for their health, those words often mean my patient has an agenda and will demand certain tests and treatments even if there is not a medical indication, even if I carefully explain to them why that is the case. This happens at least once every day."[38]

Not only are doctors' stories relating the impact of the self-diagnosis and its wobbly foundations on their personal relationships with their patients, but they are also concerned with the degree to which an accommodating, and possibly not careful enough, physician might find him or herself swept up in the unreliable self-diagnostic logic. A New Zealand doctor and his colleagues revealed a case of missed appendicitis that they attributed to the patient leading them astray: "This case is particularly pertinent as the patient, after attempting self-diagnosis consulted his family doctor. A major lesson to be learned is when formulating a differential diagnosis extreme care must be taken not to be unduly influenced by a patient's self-diagnostic conclusion."[39] Yes, the patient's proposed diagnosis plays an important part in the doctor's thinking. Eighteen per cent of diagnostic conclusions by doctors come from the diagnosis presented initially by the patient.[40]

Maybe, as Gualtieri suggests, the problem is centred in how the patient tells her diagnostic story to the doctor. Does the patient ask for a diagnosis, or ask for confirmation of their own proposed diagnosis? How that case is presented matters. Let me step back and give you a sporting analogy. Until recently in the game of rugby[41] when the referee was unsure if a try had been scored, he could turn to the television referee (who can watch a reply in slow-motion from various angles) and ask him one of two questions. He may say, "Can you see a reason *not* to award a try (touchdown)?" Or he may ask, "Try or no try?" There is a big difference between the two.[42]

In the first case, the referee is not asking the television referee to engage in independent decision making, rather he is asking him to refute the decision that a try has been scored. In the second case, he gives the television referee full authority to make the decision. Essentially, he is saying, "I couldn't see anything. I don't know. Help me out here!" To the attacking team who thinks it has scored, the first question is a relief because it implies there is a score. The second question contains no implication, and leaves the referee free to decide. The equivalent in the diagnostic setting is the self-diagnosis, where the doctor is being asked to confirm an existing opinion. Alternatively, the patient who brings symptoms, rather than a presumptive diagnosis, is giving the physician free rein to explore and define the case.[43] It is not so much that doctors are swayed by the self-diagnosis that their patients bring to the consultation room; it is more that the question is not the same and, indeed, may lead to a different outcome than if the patient presents with symptoms rather than with a candidate diagnosis.

Doctors' stories in which the patient is cast as a vulnerable and unsuspecting character, ripe for being taken advantage of by a devious commercial player proliferate. But the story of self-diagnosis is far more complex than simply that of a villainous commercial manipulator steering consumers astray. For the pharmaceutical industry to be able to promote diagnosis in view of drug sales, diagnosis has to be a phenomenon upon which a layperson would latch. But more on this later. The important thing is that doctors clearly want oversight of the sources of information to which their patients have access.

Feke's online article, referred to above, serves as an interesting case in point: "Dr. Google wants you to think he is your best friend," she writes, personifying the online presence of self-diagnostic tools in more than one way. Not only does she give him a professional title and a name, but she also instils in him desire and agency: "It can lead to people questioning their doctor's judgment even after they have been properly seen and examined," she laments, underlining the upheaval the use of online information can introduce into what she sees as a proper relationship with a diagnostic authority. She then lists the problems with the information available to patients online for working out a diagnosis on their own and concludes, "If Dr. Google were a real person, there is no question he would be sued for malpractice. He often gives inaccurate diagnoses. He promotes unnecessary testing. He causes increased worry and anxiety without a proper evaluation. He does not fulfill basic standards of care. Altogether, he breaks the tenant of medicine so graciously put forth in the Hippocratic Oath: Do no harm."

She sums up: "Take my warnings above to heart. If you have a real concern, seek out an evaluation with a medical professional. They have the training and expertise to help you on the path to health or at least a diagnosis."

A non-doctor replying under the pseudonym "Faxon" replies, "don't treat me as if I am a naughty child" and explains he would never ask for a particular treatment simply because he saw it advertised online. "Fickledame" wrote, "I would still be living in hell if it weren't for Dr Google." Another writer agreed with Feke but admonished, "I think we should all be careful to try and avoid the scolding tone with which they are presented."

As the historical review attests, quests for self-diagnosis have been going on for well over a century. Yes, industry has perhaps a wider reach now, and more tools at its disposal for communicating its messages. And yes, the public may be more uniformly schooled, or at least equipped, in the use of the media which distribute these commercial messages. But it is important to recognize that if over-diagnosis and self-diagnosis are indeed increasing trends, this is also a reflection of a cultural belief system that holds faith in diagnosis as a means of understanding the world. Seeing diagnosis as a cultural product is a recent trend. While Mildred Blaxter argued for it in the late 1970s,[44] and Phil Brown called for a sociology of diagnosis almost 20 years later,[45] it has only been in the last decade that there has been a focus on diagnosis as a topic of inquiry in and of itself.[46]

I refer to the thinking of sociologist Irving Zola for this position. When he discussed medicalization in a retrospective commentary about his earlier works, he noted that the anti-medicalization advocates who raised a clamour before he, himself, started writing about the subject, were insufficiently reflexive. His interest in the subject was something different from that of his contemporaries. They were concerned with a kind of medical imperialism (today, we might add "or industry machinations"), where doctors sat around the table, in their white lab coats, with a determined intent to usurp normal life events into their purview. Zola disagreed. For him, the problem of medicalization was one of over-reliance on the expert. It is the turning away from the doula – the experienced layperson – to look with reverence to the doctor, the lawyer, the engineer.[47] I think the same factors may be at play here in the self-diagnosis.

Yes, undoubtedly a roomful of pharmaceutical executives are sitting around a table in *Madmen* style, plotting out how to get more interest in their products. I can imagine their conversations. Somewhere someone has to ask "but what is it that people *want?*" And someone else will have to retort, "They want a sense of certainty, and of science. They want to know that what they have is real, is important. That there's a *diagnosis* for what ails them."

And this is how the pharmaceutical industry has become such a great player in the self-diagnosis business. Yes, they're plotting, but they are riding on the back of public faith in medicine. It is popular *reliance on the expert* that is at work here. When in the nineteenth century, doctors implored the public to have faith in science and to avert their gaze from the unqualified quacks, they probably did not perhaps anticipate that as they asked their patients to believe in medicine as an explanatory framework, the patients would take this commitment to science to such an extreme that they would start talking the talk themselves, rather than turning to their doctors to listen.

Owen Whooley is a medical sociologist who explains that the way medicine got its grip on professional power, climbed to the top of the hierarchy of the professions, was via the control of the episteme. To elbow out the homeopath, the hydropath, the magnetizer, and the Fletcherites, medicine got a hold of the terms of knowledge. If they could control the means by which disease was understood, the *facts* of disease, then they could control its management, its therapies, and its institutions. Diagnosis was then, and is now, vital to the episteme.[48]

The lay self-diagnosis emerges precisely from the strength of medical discourses around diagnosis, so we shouldn't be surprised at lay use of diagnosis to explain disease. Medicine has afforded such pre-eminence to diagnosis as a way of understanding what ails us, for determining the treatment, for predicting the future, and for designating the professions that we should simply expect laypeople to get their hands on diagnosis; the public have been so long indoctrinated to the importance of diagnosis that they have absorbed the lesson to a fault.

What makes this indoctrination so interesting in the context of this book is the way in which it serves as the basis for a story over which patient, doctor, and others tussle. The concern voiced by doctors is clearly over diagnosis and not anything else. It is rarely, for example, about symptoms (except in the case of medically unexplained conditions, an important exception[49]). It is sometimes about treatment, but usually only in relation to a treatment which is linked to diagnostic disagreement. No, the tension comes from how the symptoms are narrated, linked, and explained.

The location of power is under dispute precisely because of the importance assigned to diagnosis by the medical profession in its formative years and still today. While medicine instructed the public about the importance of diagnosis to gain ascendency over competing therapeutic pretendants, it probably didn't occur to them at the time, that the public would end up focusing on diagnosis to gain ascendency over medicine! As "Faxon" wrote above, she is not a naughty child; rather, like Davison's study participants, she uses the wider public knowledge to explain what afflicts her. "Faxon" wants to cast herself as the main protagonist in the story of her illness – an active agent with power to drive the narrative in the direction of her choice.

Patients' stories are important to them, but they are important to the doctor as well. We have seen how this is a point of tension, because patients are unlikely to consult a doctor if their story does not have diagnosis as a frame, yet at the same time, by appropriating diagnosis, patients step outside their authorized realm of operation. They must simultaneously believe in diagnosis but leave it in the hands of the medical professional. In the next chapter, we delve in to the stories of doctors as they narrate their role in divulging diagnosis. It's a hard task, and as they tell these stories, we learn more about what it means to be a doctor and how the profession constitutes itself via medical stories of diagnosis.

It's a hard line to hold!

CHAPTER THREE

"The Expertness of His Healer": Diagnosis, Disclosure, and the Power of a Profession

Let's return to the doctor's office from the Introduction, where the individual was waiting a bit anxiously, to hear the doctor's diagnosis. Apprehensive perhaps, but so too was the doctor, weighing up the words, thinking through how to present the case, reflecting upon the consequences of the maybe-serious diagnosis she was about to deliver. This particular diagnostic moment was nestled in as one among many in which this doctor had previously participated, and it was also for her, a moment of storytelling. On the one hand, she was preparing the story she would deliver along with the diagnosis, choosing her plot carefully, and deciding whether to cast this diagnosis as an opportunity, a lucky break, or seriously bad news. She sets the frames that shape the story and describes the potential twists. She enumerates the characters and chooses her metaphors. She would have a tale to tell the patient.

But she would also have a story to tell herself, about herself and the work she does. She might have thought to link the characters (the patient and herself) with other characters she had seen in the past, anticipating pitfalls and side stories, relying upon flashbacks to which she will need to return. The story of her work mingles with the story of the disease, its histories, legends, and fictions. Her story could be a heroic one, of tricking disease to rescue the patient, or one of despair, where the disease is an ever-present enemy, ready to strike despite her best efforts. In any case, her story is one which will imprint upon the patient, the family, the entourage, an outline which will be difficult to erase or reimagine. It creates, often inflexibly, a template for the subsequent retellings. This particular moment of storytelling is thus frequently enduring and determinant, it casts a permanent shape on the interaction, the condition, and the individuals. It is dominant.

Its power is not only contained in the blow delivered by the story's telling, if blow it will be. It is also embodied in the way it constructs the doctor, both epistemically and morally. Its impact is in the way it develops understandings – both of the patient and of the doctor – of what it means to be a doctor. Doctors' writings are replete with stories about themselves, their patients, the diagnoses they deliver, and what it means to be a doctor. The discursive construction of their stories, and of the stories told about them, are framed by the idea of *truth*. This seemingly simple term is an important anchor to the authoritative power of the diagnostic narrative.

These stories convey authority, not only to the diagnosis but also to the individual who delivers the diagnosis. Doctors become soothsayers as they provide a sense of the future. Instead of divination, however, medicine uses science to make sense of illness and does so by labelling disease, prescribing treatments, and announcing the prognosis in relation to the diagnosis. The impact of these tasks is no less great than those of the soothsayer, and Hippocrates recognized that when he described the power of the diagnosis to anchor the doctor's status: "[It will] increase his reputation as a medical practitioner."[1]

Hippocrates words suggest a calculated positioning of the doctor to achieve status. This is not generally the type of power to which I will refer in this chapter. Rather, I make reference to the place of the doctor in the social schema. I am talking about what Alfred Schofield described in 1906, the way that "a doctor is weighed in the balance as no other man is. Every act of his, every word he drops, is seed which will surely produce fruit. All he does has a double force."[2]

The power of the medical story is contained in a phenomenon Owen Whooley calls the "truth-wins-out narratives." The ascendency of medicine's knowledge over other forms of knowledge lends weight to the power of its assertions and forces assent to their models.[3] At the same time, controlling what counts as valid knowledge, even in arenas going well beyond pathophysiology,[4] the profession of medicine cements its position as the authorized diagnosis storyteller.

Still in the contemporary era, the diagnosis story continues to confirm the status of the profession (but more on that at the conclusion of this chapter). Diagnostic privilege has been something that professional groups scrap over: Who should be allowed to diagnose and in what contexts? Doctors take diagnosis very seriously as part of how they define themselves as a profession and how they view their patients. In this chapter, we look at the stories they tell about revealing a diagnosis, stories that features widely in their writings, their codes, and their protocols, and that, as I wrote above, impose a particular form on the stories others – patients, their families, the wider public – are able to tell.

We use the past as our departure point for a variety of reasons. The most important one is that it is easier to look *critically* at bygone eras, for the simple reason that we have a bit of distance. The stories and the power they convey are more visible, as they are cast in terms less familiar to us, more quaint (even though they may still follow the same or similar plot lines, as our contemporary stories). It is much harder to see this in today's material, precisely because it is closer to us.[5] But as we look at the stories associated with diagnostic delivery, I will highlight the historical to tie it in, later in the chapter, with the contemporary. What is fascinating is to see how little has actually changed, even though the trappings look so different at first glance.

I will start by pursuing the line prompted by Hippocrates's words, that is to say, to consider how the stories proposed by doctors in relation to pronouncing the diagnosis have been connected with the profession, its status, and its power. To do this, I look at the abundant works written by and to doctors discussing whether they should reveal a diagnosis to the patient. But I will also look at the stories they tell, not about themselves but about their patients and the diseases they have. By studying their stories, we can learn much about how doctors see themselves, their patients, and their competitors; their role; and the role that diagnostic knowledge played, and continues to play, in maintaining their respective standing.

This chapter presents a far-reaching survey of publications for doctors, written, for the most part, by doctors. To make this material relevant to our contemporary interest, I have started in the mid-nineteenth century at the time when scientific medicine became the status quo. My stopping point is within the lifespan of some readers, that is to say in the early 1960s, which I call the beginning of the *era of informed consent*. The move towards a systematic approach to informing patients about their condition and treatments – in fact, authorizing patients, at least in principle, to engage in medical decision making – started to gather steam in the early 1960s, moving towards generalization in the mid- to late 1970s.[6] It shifted many of the debates about telling patients what ailed them, and it also changed the details of the diagnostic stories; however, as we will see in the second half of this chapter, many stories remained the same even while the contexts shifted.

Medical power is rarely considered explicitly as such in medical writings. It is usually experienced, and expressed, rather, as a heavy burden, to be shouldered with infinite care. In a model of medical paternalism, there is a trade-off in the distribution of power. The patient must sacrifice autonomy in favour of what the doctor believes is in the patient's interests.[7]

In line with this paternalism, one of the most prevalent stories that surfaces both in historical medical writings is of the pensive and sensitive doctor heavily burdened by a knowledge he or she must share with a fragile and vulnerable patient. Typically, the patient is of a similar class to the doctor. It is rare that these stories deal with people of other classes or circumstances, except to consider them as a generic category to be dealt with rather than a subject within a specific context. As I explained in the Introduction, the stories of diagnosis are often typical for the absences which they punctuate, the voices they don't air. They are the stories of those who can afford themselves the care of a doctor and whom a doctor would be willing to attend.

Historical accounts of the poor tended to be dismissive, characterizing the patient as a different kind of patient all together, "much easier to attend to than the higher classes; their therapeutics more clearly indicated, the response of their system is generally more prompt."[8] However, the physician who wrote these words carefully advised young doctors not to shun the poor, for the benefit they could bring to a doctor's practice. They are a "potent lever to assist in establishing your professional reputation" he wrote.[9]

The typical narrative template has three protagonists: the patient (and his or her entourage), the doctor, and the disease. The careful doctor cautiously weighs up the patient's situation and character before dispensing the amount and type of information required to reduce his or her suffering. The narrative is frequently delivered as hypothetical story narrated by a sage and experienced doctor in which he makes generalizations about numerous cases he has witnessed over the course of a long career. Alternatively, the medical narrator may relate a series of individual stories in which he presents his previous successes and failures, each one in aid of whatever point he is trying to defend.[10] The latter are frequently assembled as points and counterpoints to illustrate a range of back stories and plots twists that the unwary clinician must juggle to skilfully navigate to fulfil his professional responsibilities. As he describes the patients, the narrator also ends up describing himself.

Both of these narrative styles aim to assist medical students or colleagues to deflect what my colleague Anna Jackson refers to as "death by diagnosis": a shock so great at the revelation of the disease label that the patient will expire as a result of its impact. The doctors were most concerned about what fictions a patient might generate out of the diagnostic moment, and how these could damage their spirit and hopes for cure, as I describe in this chapter. Of course, already, the notion that patients would tell themselves the wrong story was something that doctors tried valiantly to control.

John Harrison's mid-nineteenth century narratives were typical of those of many physicians for well over a century. He spoke of this most solemnly, in front of students of the Ohio Medical Lyceum, as he described delivering a diagnosis of life-threatening disease. He portrayed the patient in the most fragile of terms, and cast the doctor as having the powers both of succour and of destruction. The diagnostic moment was one at which the doctor could rescue his patient, rather than let him succumb to the diagnosis which, generally, the doctor should not announce: "Here we tread on tender ground – let us not be too sudden, or abrupt, in our communications to the sick as regards their danger," he wrote. "The voice of the physician should never be made to sound the knell of his poor suffering patient. Encouragement, not despair should be awakened by his tones, his looks, his every act and effort to rescue a sinking, trembling, dying man from the grasp of the king of terrors."[11] He recommended that the diagnosis should only ever be made to the patient when "death has set his seal on the brow, and placed his iron hand upon the heart, and the physician is called upon by the imploring demands of the patient, be not so cruel as not to deny him his last request, but in the gentlest method, make known to him his real state."[12]

It was a heavy responsibility, preserving patients from excessive fear, and was felt acutely by doctors in many eras and many settings, according to their stories. Figure 3.1 captures some of this angst on canvas. Some 60 years after Harrison's heartrending description of caring for the gravely ill, Richardson told a similar tale, but he related it in sequential details about particular patients for whom he had cared and how he had managed their cases. He reported his success as well as his failures in announcing a dreaded diagnosis, and used this score to underline, as had Harrison, the delicate path a doctor must tread. In the *St Paul Medical Journal*, writing to third-year surgical students, he also

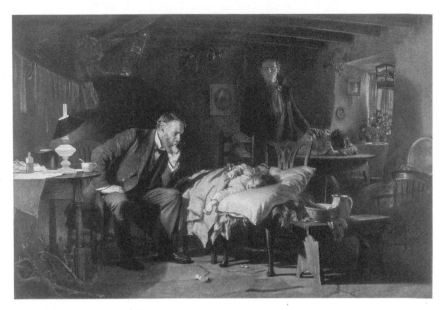

3.1 The ponderous task of diagnostic deliberation and delivery.
[Samuel Luke Fildes, Goupil, 1893. Credit: Wellcome Collection]

told of concealing a diagnosis to protect a patient from what he saw as potentially life-ending shock. Richardson believed that life was in the doctor's hands, affected by what he or she chose to say aloud.[13] Little, he explained, could compare to the "mental agony" associated with a hopeless disease. Before delineating his medical cases, he described a brave and staunch friend, a surgeon like himself, who was standing courageous, as he "descended into the valley of death." Richardson hoped that he, himself, would be able to confront his own death in due course with such serenity. However, he did not see his patients as having the same capacity.

He told, in contrast, the story of a widowed mother with malignant stomach cancer who was the sole source of support for numerous small children who, upon her death, would undoubtedly be separated and sent to "various social institutions" (one presumes, the poor house). As her surgeon, he decided that her anguish about her condition need not be amplified, as she would leave behind numerous children "friendless, fatherless and motherless."[14] On the other hand, he made a different call for a woman with breast cancer, whose children were almost independent. He revealed her diagnosis and described the likely short-term mortal outcome, "in order that she might plan her work in accordance with her time."[15] He explained that the truth "is at times hard to tell, it is a deep grief to utter it. a cruel blow to inflict it, and an awful shock to receive it." The paradox of course is that while he hoped to face his own death with equanimity, he didn't grant that same opportunity to all his patients.

Another doctor who shared these characterizations of diagnosis was Alfred T. Schofield, who told of diagnostic injury. As we saw above, he cautioned doctors that their words and acts "[have] a double force."[16] The doctor therefore had to soften the clout of his words: "And while telling no lies, [the doctor] is perfectly consistent and only telling as much of the truth as is good for his patient to know; and of this, rightly or wrongly, he must be the judge."[17]

Doctors could equally use the power of the diagnostic moment to save the patient. Revealing the diagnosis in a way that inspired hope, for example, might help the physician enlist participation in difficult treatments or prevent the spread of disease. Richardson had written that when there was hope for cure (and, particularly, if by naming the disease the patient could be scared into undergoing surgery) then the diagnosis should be given.[18] For doctor Joseph Collins the "the physician soon learns that the art of medicine consists largely in skilfully mixing falsehood and truth in order to provide the patient with an amalgam which will make the metal of life wear and keep men from being poor shrunken things, full of melancholy and indisposition, unpleasing to themselves and to those who love them."[19] Many years later Seelig echoed this advice: "The patient should *not* be told that his disease is cancer except in those uncommon instances in which special circumstances are present or in which his cooperation can be won only by telling him the nature of his disease."[20] The diagnosis could help an otherwise reluctant patient to recognize medicine's potential.

Sometimes, euphemism, rather than lying, could help create a more positive story out of the diagnostic moment. One doctor advocated telling patients about their diagnoses, but he still avoided using the word cancer: "To the layman it means almost a sentence of death, and to take away hope when we have simply removed an epithelioma is inexcusable."[21]

The skill of the physician in preserving patients from unneeded anxiety yet preparing them for their end by revealing the diagnosis was often referred to in moral terms. The duty was God-given and often conflated the use of the terms *diagnosis* and *truth*, further instilling the doctor with moral authority. This reflects Whooley's assertions about the rise of medical professionalism and ascendency being couched in narratives that force assent on the basis of what counts as factual content.[22]

These words are very important to the storyline. It's one thing to tell a patient what you think ails them; it's completely different to tell them the *truth* about their condition or to discuss their health in terms of *truth* and *lies*. Dispensing diagnosis as a truth, or a verdict (which is, etymologically, the "truth spoken," from *veir*, "true" + *dit*, "saying") is a moral, and not a clinical, stance. Referring to diagnosis as truth is to go beyond the act of communication, to assert the non-negotiable nature of the revelation. Casting the diagnosis as truth is to make no space for error or uncertainty, whether these discussions take place between doctor and patient or among colleagues. To this day, the medical subject heading (the index system for medical librarians) for discussions about the revelation of difficult or life-threatening diagnoses remains "truth disclosure."[23]

As doctors described their choices about revealing and withholding diagnosis in such moral terms, they were also able to characterize themselves as the protective guardians of the patients. When we delve, however, into their discussions of truth, we can see that they were pretty vague and, even, one could venture, self-serving (or, perhaps, we should say "practical"?) in how they defined it. What counted as true depended on the doctor's judgment. Not telling a patient a diagnosis could still be being "true to the patient," as Brown wrote.[24] He explained that "to tell *the whole truth* – that is for [the doctor's] own wisdom and discretion to judge of."[25] Similarly, Dr Worthington Hooker, from Connecticut, also told of the doctor's discretion in deciding just how much truth to dole out: "It is not to be expected of [the doctor] that he shall always tell each patient just how his case stands. His own mind is often filled with conflicting hopes and fears, and he cannot decide clearly what the probabilities are in many cases and if he thinks that he can do so, he may be very much mistaken," he wrote.[26] In support of this stance, he told about a woman who, upon learning she had arthritis, was "so frightened ... that she never returned to the orthopaedist; so convinced was she of the hopelessness of arthritis that little constructive thought was given to treatment, and within a few weeks, the nervousness resulting from her worry had quite eclipsed the trouble with her feet."[27]

Harvard professor Dr Richard Cabot was a bit of a maverick in his time, as he maintained that *telling* patients their diagnosis – telling them the "truth" – was a form of obedience to God: "God cannot lie; and man cannot work with God and lie," he wrote. In his writings, he saw diagnostic power as God given: "So man, with God's authority can take life and give life."[28] He argued that patients generally knew the truth, regardless of what was said to them, and could often see straight through any form of concealment a doctor might use. Paradoxically, however, when his own wife, Ella, faced terminal cancer, he implored her doctors not to tell her. His family maintained that his concealment of her terminal disease confirmed his "extraordinarily silly idea of telling the truth in medicine."[29] Cabot believed that he had successfully prevented her from suspecting her diagnosis, at odds with what he believed in relation to his own patients.[30]

Later publications by doctors moved away from using the word *truth* and instead talked about the diagnosis being spoken or unspoken[31] and about the patient being "told."[32] The Mayo Clinic published a collection of essays with the title *Should the Patient Be Told?*[33] punctuating the shift in location of the discussion of diagnostic disclosure from an epistemic authority and moral duty to one of communication. This is not to say, however, that the moral content of the disclosure decision disappeared.

Of course, what the doctors felt they could reveal depended on how they characterized their patients and what they thought each one could respectively handle. They told many stories about patients and patient types. Most doctors would (as had Richardson) tailor their own actions in accordance. They described a range of personality types who could or couldn't be told about a dire diagnosis. Silas Weir Mitchell wrote: "The people who really want to know if they will die of some given disease are few in number. Those who pretend they want to know are more common. Those who should not know are frequent enough, and among them one is troubled to do what seems right and to say in answer to their questions what is true."[34] He refers to this as "sick human nature"[35] and described the "nervous woman," the "hypochondriac," and the "insane" as individuals who did not need, and should not be told, the details of their diagnoses.

Dr Francis Palfrey wrote about the devastating impact of the diagnosis on the "timid and emotional" or the "weak characters liable to emotional panic and to morbid fears, and without responsibilities."[36] On the other hand, "Patients, and such friends as the patients may wish to have fully informed, are entitled to full statements of the facts of each case, provided they are of normal courage and intelligence, and are in a fit condition to receive them."[37]

More circumspect about the apparently weak, Austen Riggs wrote: "If we are to inspire courage, we must have it ourselves."[38] He cautioned that the "understanding what the significance of the patient's illness is to him ... constitutes a most important element in diagnosis ... and is absolutely indispensable to prognosis."[39] Sperry focused less on the weak than on the strong and specified that "resolute natures, in full possession of their wits, usually want to know what we think and expect and are able to 'take it.' I see no reason or warrant for withholding what we believe to be the truth from such a person ... On the other hand many persons do not even ask themselves how ill they are, let alone asking anyone else. They prefer to take what comes, as it comes. The reticence of such persons should be respected. There is no occasion and no moral obligation to intrude the supposed truth upon such minds. To do so would be a bit of gratuitous cruelty."[40] In similar tone, Maurice Davidson explained that people of a certain "mental calibre" would be relieved to know the *truth* (italics mine).[41]

The stories of diagnosis do more than just instil doctors with epistemic and moral powers and juxtapose them to particular patient personality types; they also put an important stake in the ground, constantly differentiating the scientific doctor from the unscrupulous quack, reinforcing in numerous ways the doctor as authentic and professional, esoteric and reliable, noble and discrete. Medically trained practitioners were strongly motivated to differentiate themselves from the others and wrote extensively on both the importance of, and the means by which, such differentiation could take place, including via the diagnosis. Doctors would vilify non-medical practitioners, revealing their inadequate training and unethical techniques. They would call for unity among doctors and would establish codes of ethics and associations of practitioners to create this solidarity. Diagnosis was almost a litmus test of authenticity. How a practitioner would establish a diagnosis and talk about it with the patient would helpfully distinguish the doctor from the quack.

Dr E. Graham Little explained that "the fatal weakness of the unqualified practitioner is not his lack of a medical degree, but his lack of knowledge of disease ... To contend then that the public interest can possibly be served by exempting anyone who is to enjoy the status of a registered medical practitioner, from training in those sciences by means of which alone a diagnosis of disease can be made is on the face of it is ridiculous."[42] However, it was not just the ability to diagnose that mattered; it was also the way in which diagnosis was revealed. The American Medical Association made this clear in its 1847 code of ethics: "[The physician should] … not be forward to make gloomy prognostications," in order to avoid "magnifying the importance of his services in the treatment of cure of the disease,"[43] a direct reference to quackery.

Repeatedly, the idea that only a scientifically trained and registered doctor could be trusted to give an "honest opinion" and a measured diagnosis arises in these almost fable-like tales of quackery. For example, a Dr Saundby insisted that exaggerating a diagnosis is "universally the trick of the quack, who seeks, by frightening his patient, to get him more completely in his power."[44] Drs Little and Palfrey both fed this same fire. The former maintained that only "the qualified man [is able to] interpret the signs presented by this patient, distinguish one sign from another, and to relate the signs to prognosis and treatment."[45] The latter referred to magnifying, either consciously or unconsciously, "the seriousness of their patients' conditions … [as] a heartless form of quackery."[46] Dr Johnson explained that this magnification was because "one of the earmarks of the quack is to exaggerate the gravity of a patient's condition in order to get credit for a cure that Mother Nature could have accomplished quite well unaided. It is at least absolutely dishonest, as well as cruel, thus to play on the emotions of the family"[47] What Saundby articulates most clearly among these authors is the way in which a particular posture, a restrained and discrete way of communicating about diagnosis, contributes to a doctor's success as a practitioner and to the ascendency of medicine for making sense of illness. I call what Dr Saundby is advocating an "epistemic posture." He is describing a way of behaving, a kind of comportment, which conveys knowledge and authority. Acting like a doctor is an important part of being a doctor, notably for the way in which it anchors the medical epistemic authority, or the power to control knowledge.

I opened this chapter by suggesting that history had an important contribution to make to our understanding of contemporary practice. Emily Martin has pointed out just how difficult it is to see the cultural content of contemporary practices. History, she has said, provides us with some critical distance from which to consider practices like, in this case, telling stories about diagnosis.[48]

This little journey into the past has highlighted some important motifs that are produced by diagnosis and by doctors' stories about the diagnostic moment. It has emphasized how duty and control interact and how this influences what stories can be told. While the words I have shared above may seem particularly old world to a reader in the twenty-first century, the ideas and values they capture and the purposes they serve are not completely unfamiliar. There is a growing storytelling corps of physicians in our contemporary world. From TV doctors to online blogs and doctor-authored trade books about disease, there are many ways in which doctors' stories about diagnosis circulate in our consciousness.

Not all of these works are self-consciously about storytelling, but Lisa Sanders's *Every Patient Tells a Story* clearly is. The purpose of her book is to highlight diagnosis, what she calls "this crucial linchpin of medicine."[49] By framing it as crucial, Sanders is underlining one more time (in case we needed to be reminded) how pivotal diagnosis is. It is critical, indispensable, the pivot upon which everything is exquisitely balanced. She confers upon diagnosis, in casting it thus, an immense part in the drama of illness.

But in addition to its mechanisms of power, diagnosis itself is for Sanders, a story. It is the same story that we've discussed before, which links clues and twists, fitting things together so that they make sense. The diagnostic story is also its own reward. It can be entertaining, pedagogical, and simply entertaining: "Doctors take pleasure in recounting the completed story of their complex diagnoses."

Sanders celebrates diagnosis – it represents a better understanding of illness and leads to better therapies. It's also an art, which depends on a curious, stubborn, critical doctor-detective being able to put the pieces together into a logical narrative. The clues are always in the story: the patient's as well as the doctor's. In so doing, she extols the diagnosis, revealing its importance.

She describes doctors listening carefully to patient stories and then looking for the interface between an experiential tale and one that can be told in diagnosis. The epiphany of diagnosis, for the doctor, is not the epiphany of crisis that the patient experiences upon being told of a life-threatening diagnosis; it is, for the doctor, the moment where he or she knows what and if medicine can offer anything in the way of succour.

What is the metanarrative that Sanders is sharing with us in this book? She is demonstrating the simultaneous burden and promise of diagnosis. While we can see diagnostic authority as wielding power, Sanders shows how the truth of diagnosis is shrouded in uncertainty but also in fascination. It is an unwieldy, yet esoteric power. It is a puzzle that often looks straightforward but is also often fraught with obstacles. She maintains a faith in (and indeed celebrates!) the scientifically developed skills of medicine.

In this era of consent medicine, where sharing the diagnosis with the patient has become an expectation rather than a point of grand debate, Sanders's focus is less on the way that a diagnosis is delivered and its impact, and more on the way that stories from the patient and from the doctor contribute to the important task of diagnosis. She reminds us that William Osler, the first physician-in-chief at Johns Hopkins and author of the seminal *The Principles and Practice of Medicine*, instructed his trainees that it was more important to know "what kind of patient has the disease, than what sort of disease that person has,"[50] and she takes this to mean that understanding the stories of the patient will help lead doctors to their position about what ails the patient and what therapeutic assistance they can bring to the case.

She describes how the patient and the diagnostician share their stories. We discussed this in another form in relation to Michael Balint's theories in the previous chapter where he described diagnosis operating in proposals and counterproposals floating back and forth between the layperson and the doctor. Sanders confirms in unambiguous terms how the power of the profession is exercised via the stories it is able to construct from the diagnostic process.

"What the physician brings," she writes "is the knowledge and understanding that will help him order that story so that it makes sense both to the doctor – who uses it to make diagnosis – and to the patient – who must then incorporate that subplot into the larger story of his life."[51] Even while she has described the diagnostic process in terms of collaboration, comparing it to a shared authorship where two writers would keep exchanging drafts of the story, she still leaves the framing to the doctor, who will ground the plot in the power of diagnosis.

I am not using Sanders's words to condemn either medicine or Sanders herself for holding, believing in, or imposing the framing mechanism. Rather, I am observing this in order to provide a better understanding of diagnosis's implicit power to transform and shift the personal stories of patients. This is part of a bigger story, one which places the "expert" at the heart of the understanding of human existence (as I described Zola doing in his discussions of medicalization).

There may be instances of "bad guys in white coats" using their medical status to unleash their demons, and upset people's lives, but that's not the point.

The point is, as Sanders has said most eloquently: Diagnosis counts. It is an important medical tool that results from, and generates new, stories and tales. Without diagnosis, and its narrative capacity, as Sanders clearly demonstrates, people would die.

Siddartha Mukherjee has written the book that always should have been written, one that combines historical, clinical, genetic, poetic, and philosophical reflections on the dread disease(s) we call cancer.[52] *The Emperor of All Maladies* was Mukherjee's first book, and it won the Pulitzer Prize for non-fiction. It is a masterful, readable, and hefty tome. Mukherjee is a haematology-oncologist who works and teaches at Columbia University. He, like Sanders, writes a bit of a detective story, as he discusses one of today's most dreaded diagnoses. He explains the trails and the false trails that science and medicine have taken to understand, and perhaps one day cure, cancer in many of its forms.

Mukherjee, in the tradition of many of the historical doctor-writers we reviewed in the previous chapter, is a master of narrative, as he weaves together cases, historical data, and personal musings to draw a portrait of what he calls *The Emperor of All Maladies*. This is a braided (auto)biography featuring three prominent sets of characters with their individual narratives: the patients, the doctor, and the diseases. Yet within each strand is an array of subplots and backstories that Mukherjee may argue are about cancer, but that are, to this reader at least, clearly about Mukherjee himself and his relation to his specialization in cancer medicine.

What Mukherjee achieves through this form of narration is a transformation of a historical chronicle into an embodied story. If we recall Fludernik's definition of storytelling, then to be a narrative, the story needs to be personified, or told through individual subjects.[53] Mukherjee's patient stories provide a powerful means by which to turn the story of cancer into a riveting narrative: "On the morning of May 19, 2004, Carla Reed, a thirty-year-old kindergarten teacher ..." starts Mukherjee, in the first sentence of his book, launching into the patient story that will weave itself in his own narrative until the end. Carla Reed will soon learn that she has leukaemia, and Mukherjee will follow her until her total remission some five years later. There will be other patient stories, briefly told – of young Steve Harmon who will die of oesophageal cancer despite valiant treatment, of elderly Beatrice Sorenson whose pancreatic cancer will put an end to her days – but there will only be a few patients, like Carla, whose narratives we will follow from beginning to what looks like successful end.

One of them is the athlete Ben Orman, who will recover from his Hodgkin's lymphoma, and another is Kate Fitz, a 66-year-old woman with a large lung mass. Mukherjee describes how he revealed the diagnosis to Ben Orman: "I watched the thought pick up velocity in his brain, until it had reached its full impact. 'It's going to be a long haul. A marathon,' I stammered apologetically, groping for an analogy. 'But we'll get to the end.' He nodded again silently, as if he already knew."[54]

Kate Fitz, on the other hand, was not Mukherjee's patient, and he describes the diagnostic moment from the perspective of an observer. During his oncology fellowship, he works with Thomas Lynch, a lung cancer doctor. "I was about to enter the room," wrote Mukherjee, "when Lynch caught me by the shoulder and pulled me into the side room. He had looked through her scan and her reports ... but more important, he had seen Fitz folded over in fear in the waiting room. Right now, he said, she needed something else. 'Resuscitation,' he called it cryptically as he strode into her room."[55]

What Lynch means by resuscitation is a kind of moral recovery, aimed at assisting patients to reconcile themselves with death, at the same time, it is, according to Mukherjee, an opportunity to wrest the control of his patients' imagination from death (we will read more about the personification of death in chapter 4, the diagnostic moment in fiction). What Mukherjee observes in his mentor is the way Lynch emphasizes what he will do, rather than what the outcomes will be. He explains relapse as something "we will tend to when that happens."[56] He finds out more about what matters in Fitz's life. He "repossesses" her imagination. However, Kate Fitz will live beyond all expectations.

Of the three patients whose stories Mukherjee relates, all have a life beyond cancer. Orman's story becomes iconic: "Orman epitomized the afterlife of cancer – eager to forget the clinic and its bleak rituals, like a bad trip to a foreign country."[57] Fitz becomes able to "see" forward, "effervescence pour[ing] out of every spigot of her soul."[58] And Carla is still in remission, five years after the diagnostic announcement that Mukherjee thought would end in death.

Mukherjee's patient stories of diagnosis serve a number of functions. They enable him to tell his broader story, one of coming of age as a cancer specialist in an era where there are so many signs of promise, and yet so many disappointments. He could have simply written a literature review, or a disease history, but neither would have had anywhere near the impact or the ability to draw in readers in the way that his narrative clearly does. It's a *New Yorker* style account, where every player is described physically, even if only from a grainy historical photograph; these patients become real to us, no matter that we've never met them.

He calls these three patients a "routine spectrum of survivors,"[59] and he provides them as a way of making oncology and cancer survivorship meaningful concepts: "It is an old complaint about the practice of medicine that it inures you to the idea of death. But, when medicine inures you to the idea of life, to survival, then it has failed utterly ... but surely, it was the most sublime moment of my clinical life to have watched that voyage in reverse, to encounter men and women *returning* from the strange country – to see them so very close, clambering back."[60] By telling these stories, albeit among others with less favourable outcomes, Mukherjee gives his readers a reason to hope and a reason to believe in the possibility of Mukherjee's medicine.

Ranjana Srivastava is also an oncologist. Her book is entitled *Tell Me the Truth: Conversations about Life and Death*.[61] This little book has numerous stand-alone stories about patients Srivastava has looked after and her interactions with them. The cover image, rather than medical iconography, shows a cup of tea and a saucer. And in line with this image of folk comfort and domesticity, this book is not really about medicine. While it is written by a doctor, and tells stories that only a doctor could tell, its stories nibble away at the powerful medicine that Sanders and Mukherjee write about. Srivastava's patients are the protagonists in this tale.

Srivastava starts her story in her childhood. She recalls the death of her beloved grandmother, who went from exceptional good health to declining dramatically to her death in a matter of weeks. As a little girl, she was traumatized by this unexpected transformation. As a practising oncologist, she reinterprets this difficult phase in her life and that of her family as one in which medicine failed to deliver on its promises.

"It took weeks, maybe months, to diagnose the condition, and when the diagnosis was made, it was one whose very name filled the mind with a sense of unfathomable foreboding and unending sorrow"[62] she remembers. She then proceeds to draw parallels between what she recalls of her grandmother's death and what she observes in her contemporary patients. As she does so, there is a tension in her writing about the importance of diagnosis and its simultaneous insignificance. She is constantly underlining how diagnosis makes the doctor and is everything to the patient, and just as quickly pushes those beliefs away to explain how the focus on the diagnosis restricts the emotional and professional experience of doctoring. She puts diagnosis in a backseat despite at the same time using it as the primary framing device.

For example, Srivastava thinks critically about the emphasis on diagnosis in the training of doctors. "I reflect how partial doctors are to terms such as 'fix,' 'cure,' and 'conquer'" she writes. "The medical student counts a successful rotation as one with procedures. How many intravenous lines or chest tubes did she get to watch? Did anyone let her do any simple tasks? The resident and registrar are triumphant when they clinch a diagnosis ... absent from this narrative of professional development is a cohesive way to deal with ... the plethora of emotions that accompany our perceived failure at conquering disease and suffering."[63]

And yet at the same time, she proclaims that "these are exciting times in medicine," underlining the importance of diagnosis, therapy and science. See-sawing back again, practically in the next breath, she refutes the power of oncology: "I also keep hoping that I never lose sight of the fact that no therapeutic discovery will ever dispense with the need for good judgement, sensitive communication and the art of letting go."[64]

Mingled among the stories of her patients, she tells stories about her friends, herself and her family, as they learn of, or experience, dire diagnoses of cancer and other disorders. Here again, she underlines the power of diagnosis, then quickly shifts her gaze towards non-diagnostic priorities. Discussing her mother's illness, she explained, "it wasn't the doctors' lack of knowledge but a lapse in its application somewhere that debilitated and nearly killed her. Since no firm diagnosis was ever reached, there was no specific treatment either."[65] That hardly mattered, however, given that her mother's cure came from completely outside of medicine. It was a man with no formal qualifications, one who she described as "being part doctor, part pharmacist, part folk-healer; a man who had 'compounded' the skills he had picked up from observing the professionals,"[66] to whom Srivastava attributes her mother's cure. It was his interest in her mother's welfare that helped her to recover. Who needs medicine, then? one might be prompted to ask.

Srivastava's hope niches, unlike Mukherjee's, not in the power of science, rather in the resources of humanity. She writes about how the telling a patient they have cancer for the first time "is the first fall of the oncologist's gavel in a patient's life"[67] but also muses that "it often takes the diagnosis of a dire illness for them to re-evaluate their life and place the small things in perspective."[68]

Rather than present the readers with a heroic vision of medicine, Srivastava exposes her readers to a heroic view of cancer patients. She barely mentions the chemotherapy regimens and the careful adjustment of protocols that she undertakes in relation to falling blood counts, opportunistic infections, or unexpected metastases – highly technical and skilled decisions she must make on a daily basis as a medical oncologist – she explores the characters and reactions of individual patients facing the life-altering diagnoses she dishes out.

Just as she starts her story in her childhood experience, she finishes it in her own personal thoughts about life and death: "The single most important thing that I have learnt from being an oncologist is to be grateful. I am simply grateful for my life and my health."[69] She maintains faith in medicine and its power, but also in the patient's perspective of life itself.

Whether in the past or the present, there are important similarities between these stories by doctors which discuss the revelation of the diagnosis to the patient. Even in seemingly contradictory tales, like Srivastava's, where she recounts the doctor taking the back seat to the patient, Schofields idea about the doctor's "double force" is confirmed in enduring ways. The "gavel" Srivastava describes is not different from Mukherjee's "resuscitation" and Harrison's 1844 "effort to rescue [the] sinking, trembling, dying man." They are words, yes, but terribly powerful ones, just as able to sink the patient as to rescue her. The treatment of the diagnostic pronouncement transcends its historical context and continues to resonate in contemporary diagnosis stories.

Diagnosis today continues to confirm medical authority as it did in Hippocratic times and in the historical material reviewed above. Not only does the pursuit of the diagnosis construct the patient-doctor relationship, but it still differentiates doctor from other health professionals and professional from lay. Diagnosis still serves as a way of deflecting threats to medical authority.

While the threats to modern medicine are not identical to those in the nineteenth century, neither are they totally different. A number of professions (nurse practitioner, physiotherapist) make forays into diagnosis, and while these diagnosticians are not put into the same category as the last-century quack, their diagnostic incursions are strictly enforced and monitored by the medical profession. In many jurisdictions, where diagnosis can be performed by other professions than medicine, it is allowed only in medically supervised settings. The entry into practice and the diagnostic scope of non-doctor diagnosticians is limited: approved and monitored by the medical profession.

However, the esoteric nature of diagnosis remains enticing, and being able to think "like a doctor" is a valued attribute. It is the title of Lisa Sanders's popular *New York Times* column and upcoming Netflix series, which challenge laypeople to name peculiar presentations of disease. Similarly, as the succeeding chapters in this book emphasize, this way of thinking features prominently in many aspects of popular culture like TV shows, movies, novels, and cartoons.

What I want to underline most vividly in this chapter is the way in which diagnosis *makes* a profession and the role that truth plays in this professional construction. Few doctors would dispute the first point of the previous sentence. The professional *still* differentiates herself from the layperson by virtue of diagnosis; the pursuit of the diagnosis is usually what leads a patient to consult in the first place. Diagnosis still embodies truth via its commitment to science and to an evidence base. It continues to differentiate the doctor from the non-scientific practitioner or from other practitioners (non-scientific, nursing, osteopathic, and so forth).

A Foucauldian analysis of the discursive position of truth in diagnosis stories would underline how it constructs a regime of power. For Foucault, truth is power and the truth orientation in these diagnosis stories follows at least four of the traits he maintains characterize regimes of truth. The medical truth is framed by medicine's own scientific discourse. It is a truth which society demands, as there are ever-clamouring voices for scientific explanations of the conditions which ail us. It circulates pervasively (as this book describes), and it is produced under the control of the dominant social apparatus of medicine.[70]

In addition to creating truth, diagnosis creates a social need and social consequences, for patient and doctor alike. This further explains medicine's concern with diagnostic disclosure and its modalities. Particularly when the outcome of the diagnosis is beyond the diagnoser's control, as is often the case with the dire diagnosis, the focus may shift from the disease process to the means by which the diagnosis is delivered. Putting a name to a disease remains transformative for the individual who receives a substantial diagnosis. Naming it emerges from, and contributes to, the authority of the medical profession in contemporary society. Friedson explained this in sociological terms: "Where illness is the ubiquitous label for deviance in an age, the profession that is custodian of the label is ascendant,"[71] and the importance of this role is validated not only by the doctor's knowledge of diagnosis and disease but also by the manner in which he or she tells the diagnostic story.

Like duelling banjos, the patient and the diagnostician pick up refrains from each other, each time echoing but adding. However, in these medical renditions of the roles expected of each player, there are expectations about who tells whom what that tell a story about what it is to be a professional doctor. Patients are supposed to tell all in relation to what ails them (as long as it isn't pre-shaped by Dr Google), while the doctor gets to decide what information is germane. This is more than (but of course includes) a simple paternalistic approach to the individual patient; it is a discretionary approach that brings a different way of thinking about information, of navigating the morass of direct-to-patient communication, but that also protects the esoteric nature of information held by the members of the profession.

While doctors were concerned about quacks exercising power upon the patients and their families via diagnosis, they did not necessarily consider their own exercise of power. Cabot was one prominent counter-example. He maintained that it had an important place in formal medical settings. He used it to confirm the authority of the registered medical professional, both in reference to the unqualified practitioner and in reference to the layperson. At the time he wrote, the gap between professional and lay understandings of diagnosis was widening as diagnostic technologies developed and the emphasis on diagnosis in private practice developed. But diagnosis was, in his view, central to medical authority. Clear and correctly arrived at diagnoses would reduce the commercial promotion of therapeutics by unqualified practitioners. Cabot argued vehemently, however, that patients were capable of, and should be entitled to, the name of their disease. He engaged in frank written, and one presumes, verbal debates with his patients about what ailed them.[72]

These debates between patient and doctor laid down the parameters of both lay and professional roles and were pivotal in empowering the layperson as well. One seminal analysis of diagnostic debates was written in the 1960s by psychiatrist Michael Balint, whom we touched on briefly earlier. He organized observational study groups to try to understand the doctor-patient relationship and its impact on patient outcomes. His first thesis was that patients presented their symptoms *as* diagnoses, negotiating and bartering with the doctor until such time as the diagnosis proposed by the doctor as an explanation for the symptoms resonated enough with patients that they were able to accept the formal medical diagnosis as probable and plausible: "The variety of illnesses available to any one individual is limited by his constitution, up-bringing, social position, his conscious or unconscious fears and fantasies about illnesses, etc."[73] According to Balint, the negotiating around diagnosis played an important role in "settling a patient who cannot get completely cured in an acceptable illness."[74] This involves proposing, counter-proposing, and compromising so that the dysfunction is organized; the patient will be able to express her problems, the therapy is rational, and cure (if possible) is achieved.

This is where Balint emphasized the importance of the diagnostic naming. "Finding 'nothing wrong' is no answer to the patient's most burning demand, for a demand for a name for his illness. Apart from the almost universal fear that what we have found is so frightening that we will not tell him, he feels that 'nothing wrong' means only that we have not found out and therefore cannot tell him what it is that frightens or worries him and causes him pain ... It would certainly be no help to him to know ... that the statement 'nothing wrong' sometimes really means that medicine does not know what is wrong in his particular case."[75]

Balint's book was clearly written for doctors to help them manage the sometimes-problematic relationships they endured with their patients. Already, the possessive pronoun used to characterize the patient ("his") as opposed to an autonomous non-specific article ("the") indicates the extension of professional authority.

But, finally, we can't overlook the authority which results from, as underlined by the words of Hippocrates in the Introduction, the ability to "say what is going to happen." Any discussion of diagnostic revelation must acknowledge the presumed link to prognosis that a particular diagnosis can suggest. As certain as a doctor may be about a diagnosis, prognosis will remain, however, an uncertain affair and will require the doctor to try to sort out and untangle probabilities and possibilities. At the same time, this uncertain prognostication will end up being one more example of the exercise of power. Philosopher and oncologist Antonella Surbone describes this as an asymmetry, a reinforcing of power imbalance between patient and doctor:

> By reciting survival statistics in front of our patients, rather than contributing to their self-determination, we most often acquire a tremendous power. The power that modern medicine seems to have lost in terms of how the figure of the physician is perceived (no longer a god), we re-establish through our easily pronouncing life and death sentences. Diagnosis and prognosis are formidable tools indeed, and the magic can continue.[76]

While many of these authors are reluctant to venture into prognosis on the basis of the diagnosis proffered, by mentioning the diagnosis, a number of undesirable outcomes become manifest and mandate that the doctor either "conceal ... the danger of death"[77] or alternatively "discharge his duty, painful and heart-rending though it be."[78]

As we tie up this chapter, it's pretty clear that having the last word in the story of diagnosis is, to use Surbone's words, a formidable thing. Regardless of how an individual doctor might narrate diagnosis in the one-on-one setting, the collective recognition of the role of medicine in untangling the mysteries of life is undeniable. It is part of what Blaxter (whose words we will encounter in greater depth in chapter 7) refers to as complex systems that "control both medical practice and the patient's medical experience."[79] This is a system that puts diagnosis at its centre and the doctor at the helm.

CHAPTER FOUR

"The News Is Not Altogether Comforting": Fiction and the Diagnostic Moment

We've talked about how diagnosis *is* one kind of narrative, connecting symptoms into a plausible explanation with a beginning, a middle, and maybe an end. But diagnosis is also *contained* in narrative. It figures prominently in fiction, and exercises power there as well. In fiction, the diagnosis is always an impetus for transformation, a mechanism via which the characters can reveal themselves, a launching pad for reactions, responses, and actions. Diagnosis in fiction is never accidental. It serves a fundamental purpose when it surfaces. But the way it works in fiction is not necessarily a reflection of how it works in real life. It is a creation, a representation: albeit a frequent one.

I love to read. This doesn't mean that I have my nose buried in weighty academic tomes or technical journal articles. I love to read mysteries, crime thrillers, contemporary, and classic literature. What matters to me is the plot. There needs to be a good storyline to keep me enthralled. My thought processes work very quickly, and without a plot to anchor me, I lose interest quickly. As I was writing my first diagnosis book, I was sifting about, looking for an epigraph to one of my chapters. I wanted something beautifully written; using I-am-not-sure-which medical humanities database, I put in the word *diagnosis*. Lazily, I selected one or two entries that were connected to a free online full text service, and I started to read Ian McEwan's *Saturday*.[1] This classic McEwan narrated a Saturday morning in the life of a neurosurgeon off-call. Lots of things happen on this Saturday, but the description of one event in particular was to become my epigraph.

The neurosurgeon (Perowne, as it happens) was driving to the market and rear-ended the car in front of him. The occupants of the car, most unfortunately, were thugs, and

> they stormed out of the car ready to rough him up. Perowne wasn't sure how he was going to find his way out of trouble. There were three of them, and only one of him. And, while he prepared to defend himself, and looked at the gang leader, in the mind of the neurosurgeon facing getting thumped "there remains in a portion of his thoughts a droning, pedestrian diagnostician who notes poor self-control, emotional lability, explosive temper, suggestive of reduced levels of GABA among the appropriate binding sites on striatal neurons."[2]

"Your father had it. Now you've got it too,"[3] he said out loud to the gang leader, making an implicit reference to Huntington's disease, the diagnosis associated with the symptoms he noted above. Perowne's sidewalk diagnosis, delivered as if "by a witch doctor delivering a curse,"[4] immediately disarmed Baxter. The two men were extracted, by these words, from the violent confrontation, as the diagnosis shifted the locus of control and the stakes: "When you are diseased it is unwise to abuse the shaman."[5] Baxter calls off his men; the moment is averted (even though there are more moments to come).

McEwan is not a neurosurgeon himself, but to do his research for this book, he shadowed consultant neurosurgeon Neil Kitchen for months. He described diagnosis as if from the eyes of a specialist diagnostician, casting himself as half magician, half technician.

Saturday brought to my attention what I am calling the *diagnosis novel*: a work of literature which uses diagnosis and the diagnostic moment in a prominent way in a work of fiction. I was fascinated that such a genre existed and wondered how to find more examples. "You talk about it with people around you," advised a colleague from the English department. "Get the word out."

However, there was no real need to get the word out. Diagnosis novels just kept falling into my lap. Every new book that I came by would use diagnosis as the device around which the narrative or characters would pivot: the book I picked up in a giveaway pile in North Beverly, Massachusetts; the two books (thrillers) I bought in the airport before a long-haul trip; the first book on the stack my colleague at Exeter showed me on the guest room dresser saying, "if you need anything to read"; the pile of young adult books my granddaughter was reading for summer holidays ...

The uses authors make of diagnosis are many and varied. In some cases, it is the disease and in others it is the diagnosis which serves as a trigger for the narrative. In others (*Saturday* being a prime example), diagnosis is a device to arm a doctor with tangible power to shift the direction of particular activities. Yet in a different example, the diagnosis empties the doctor of any power at all (it is death that has power and diagnosis that is simply an illusion of power). In this chapter, I describe a sample of diagnosis novels that make influential use of the moment of disclosure.

I will start with a novel that uses diagnosis as a trigger to frame the narrative. The particularly moving case in point is Australian Anna Funder's *All That I Am*.[6] This novel takes diagnosis from the perspective of the one who receives, rather than delivers, a diagnosis. It recounts the tale of the narrator's cousin as a Nazi resistant via memories that are allowed to emerge, paradoxically, as a result of the diagnosis of Alzheimer's disease, a disease usually associated with memory loss, not retrieval:

> "I am afraid, Mrs Becker, the news is not altogether comforting."
> I am in a posh private clinic in Bondi Junction with harbour views. Professor Melnikoff has silver hair and half-glasses, a sky-blue silk tie, and long hands clasped together on his desk. His thumbs play drily with one another. I wonder whether this man has been trained to deal with the people *around* the body part of interest to him, in this case, my brain ...
> ... And he has seen inside my mind; he is preparing to tell me the shape and weight and creeping betrayals of it ... "It's *Doctor* Becker actually."[7]

The doctor explains:

> "It's the beginning of deficit accumulation – aphasia, short-term memory loss, perhaps damage to some aspects of spatial awareness to judge from the location of the plaquing." He points to soupy areas at the upper front part of my brain. "Possibly some effect on your sight, but let's hope not at this stage." ...

"Actually, Professor, I am remembering more, not less."[8]

The doctor is baffled and explains: "Some research suggests that more vivid long-term recollections are thrown up as the short-term memory deteriorates. Occasionally, intense epiphenomena may be experienced by people who are in danger of losing their sight. These are hypotheses.

No more."[9] However, for Ruth Wesemann, who receives this diagnosis, the ability to return to her long-term recollections enables her to return to, and recount, an important chapter in her life.

Her memories take her back to war-time Europe and to her cousin Dora Fabian, a fellow political refugee and Jewish resistant. The book weaves together two versions of Dora's story: Ruth's, told years after Dora's presumed murder, and the tale told by her sometimes lover, and fellow political exile, Ernst Toller, an author and a playwright who drafts his tale in the immediate period after Dora's death. He sought refuge in New York and is trying to tell her story before he commits suicide. He writes to remember her, while Ruth remembers via diagnosis. Both approaches are damned.

As Toller writes, "The act of remembering Dora did bring her back ... now that I have summoned her up and written her down, she is more dead than before."[10] He will follow her in death as he has attempted to follow-lead her politically in his attempt to decry the Hitler regime. But he has "failed" her, as has Ruth. Toller fails her by being unable to prevent Dora's death from being seen as suicide. Ruth has failed her by association. Her husband, Hans, has turned informant and has literally damned the cause.

Not only do the two stories jostle and jockey as they piece together the Dora's story, but Ruth's chapters also jostle among themselves. Her diagnosis allows her to navigate freely between her present and her past. She does so by alternating between her current life and her memories, and savours the chaos of fact and fiction, of memory and present. As her health deteriorates, she falls and breaks her hip. While hospitalized, she takes pethidine for pain which reinforces her memory's back and forth:

> They have added something to the drip. it is collapsing time. I see things I have imagined so many times that they are fact to me. And other things I have known without seeing ... Memory has its own ideas; it snatches elements of story from whenever, tries to put them together. It comes back at you from all angles, with all that you later knew, and it gives you the news.[11]

The more Ruth's brain is addled – be it by the neurofibrillary tangles of Alzheimer's disease or by pethidine – the closer she gets to being able to tell the truth of her cousin's sacrifice, and she clings to this ability. When visited by the resident, he suggests she take a mild antipsychotic.

> "I am not hallucinating."
> "No. No, well. It's entirely up to you."
> But that's the thing, boyo, it's *not*. This vast life – the real, interior one in which we remain linked to the dead (because the dream inside us ignores trivialities like breath, or absence) – this vast life is *not* under our control.[12]

Ruth reimagines a life for Dora and tries to give her another life, "one with a different ending." She explains that "the human brain cannot encompass total absence. Like infinity, it is simply not something that the organ runs to. The space someone leaves must be filled, so we dream forever of those who are no longer here. Our minds make them live again."[13]

> But Alzheimer's *Gott sei dank*, is not what I've got. It's just that occasionally, as on the edge of sleep, an obscure memory pops up, like a slide in a carousel.[14]

The young adult novel *Alone on a Wide, Wide Sea* by Michael Morpurgo also uses diagnosis as a narrative trigger for a fictional memoire.[15] It depicts the story of the rather tragic life of Arthur Hobhouse, one of the sad English World War II orphan migrants to Australia. After the death of his parents during a bombing raid in London, Arthur is first sent to an orphanage and then packed off to Australia, where he hopes he will find a new family. Instead, he finds himself in an outback station where Mr Bacon, the owner of Cooper's Station, kept ten young children in deplorable conditions. Arthur's life quickly turns to one of burden and deprivation. He tries to hang on to his past, and he thinks he remembers taking leave of an older sister as he embarked for Australia. He doesn't know if this memory is real, but the point of his story is to dig deep into his past to figure that out.

> The earliest memories I have are all confused somehow, and out of focus. For instance, I've always known I had a sister, an older sister. All my life she's been somewhere in the deepest recesses either of my memory or my

imagination – sometimes I can't really be sure which – and she was called Kitty. When they sent me away, she wasn't with me. I wish I knew why. I try to picture her, and sometimes I can. I see a pale delicate face with deep dark eyes that are filled with tears. She is giving me a small key, but I don't remember what the key is for. It's on a piece of string. She hangs it around my neck, and tells me I'm to wear it always."[16]

To tell a story, Arthur puts, one needs a starting point, and he simply doesn't have one. He can't check to see if his memories are shared by anyone else, so he has no beginning. He explains, "I should start at the beginning, I know that. But the trouble is that I don't know the beginning. I wish I did."[17] He continues, "They say you can't begin a story without knowing the end. Until recently I didn't know the end, but now I do. So I can begin, and I'll begin from the very first day I can be sure I remember."[18] By "knowing the end" Arthur is referring to his own diagnosis, which he reports in the late chapters of the book.

That evening as we celebrated [the launch of the boat he designed, built, and named after his sister, Kitty] I knew something wasn't quite right. I felt dizzy first, then there was a pain in my head that wouldn't go away. I'd always felt fit as a fiddle before, so when I fainted the next morning Zita called the doctor. So the saga began – the tests, the waiting, more tests, more waiting, then the results, the verdict. The doctor gave it to me straight, because I asked him to. I had a brain tumour – malignant, advanced, aggressive. There was nothing they could do … when I asked how long I'd got, he said, "Months."

"How many?"

"Five or six, difficult to be precise about it. I'm sorry."

"So am I," I said.[19]

It is this diagnostic moment, the "end" that inspires Arthur to tell his story. He recounts his escape from Mr Bacon's compound with his good friend Marty and his sanctuary with an eccentric middle-aged widow, who provides temporary homes for wallabies, kangaroo joeys who have lost their mothers, and all form of "waifs" and "strays."[20] He explains how he learned how to build boats, worked in the mines, considered suicide, and finally fell in love with and married one of his nurses. He has a daughter, who, after his death, sails solo to England to look for Kitty on a boat Arthur made with her. The daughter's saga on the wide, wide sea provides a classic coming of age story that results not only in her transition to adulthood but also in the completion of her father's story.

Arthur Hailey is well known for his procedural novels. Whether it be landing an airplane or unpacking the politics of the automobile industry, his novels place the protagonist in a highly specialized arena that provides a point of breathless attention for his readers. His 1959 novel *The Final Diagnosis* places the drama in the medical setting and uses diagnosis to underline every stake or play for power in an action-filled, yet struggling, regional hospital.[21] This novel, which will remind contemporary readers of *Grey's Anatomy*, a kind of soap opera told through the stories of doctors and their foibles, is a lively story about relationships and their dysfunctions. Diagnosis is the mechanism by which power and prestige are negotiated and distributed, the righteous are rewarded, and the evil are punished. Those who are diagnosed, as well as those who diagnose, jostle among one another and find themselves at different times on either end of the diagnostic announcement.

Diagnosis is everywhere at Three Counties Hospital and throughout the novel is cast as an emerging symbol of modern clinical practice. From a run-down organization managed by "doddering incompetents,"[22] its new medical director tightened up the operations, replaced staff, and transformed the hospital's administration. Diagnosis is at the heart of the transformation, as it is the tension around who controls diagnosis that drives the story. At Three Counties, various teams of doctors make presumptive diagnoses for which they then require the confirmation of the pathologist. From screening to post-mortem, the laboratory of Dr Joe Pearson makes the ultimate diagnosis, settles on the final verdict. As Pearson himself explains to a group of first-year nursing students, the pathologist is "the doctor the patient seldom sees. Yet few departments of a hospital have more effect on a patient's welfare." He continues: "It is pathology which tests a patient's blood, checks his excrements, tracks down his diseases, decides whether his tumor is malignant or benign. It is pathology which advises the patients' physician on disease and sometimes, when all else in medicine fails … it is the pathologist who makes the final diagnosis."[23]

The power of the pathologist is made salient in the regular surgical mortality meeting, where patient deaths are reviewed. At these meetings, the other medical staff wait with bated breath to hear whether their own diagnoses of the patients who died were correct: "It was an ordeal for anyone to describe their diagnosis and treatment of a patient who had died, then have others give their opinion, and finally the pathologist report his findings from the autopsy, and Joe Pearson never spared anyone."[24]

Despite the importance of his role, the aging and cantankerous Pearson is a vestige of the previous administration and he fails to ensure the rigour of his diagnoses, an error that will ultimately lead to his demise. While he comes up short on a number of fronts (general modernization, tracking routine testing), it is the missed diagnoses that cost Pearson his job. On the one hand, he fails to test properly for rhesus (blood type) incompatibility in a pregnant woman, which leads to the death of her premature infant. This is in spite of the fact that the father of the infant, who is a technician in Pearson's lab, points out that a more modern test is available for blood typing before his baby's death. Upon making this observation, he is lambasted for insubordination. On the other hand, Pearson does not keep up with routine testing for communicable diseases in new dietary department staff, which result in a typhoid epidemic that almost closes the hospital.

Pearson steps down in disgrace, and his lab technician who identifies the food worker who is carrying and spreading typhoid wins a scholarship to medical school. In *The Final Diagnosis*, diagnostic power generates social power in the hospital. In the background of these two events is yet another diagnostic story. A young nurse, in love with one of the surgical residents, receives the diagnosis of malignant osteosarcoma. This, Pearson diagnoses correctly. And even though this subplot, a love interest, pales in significance to the other two, it serves to punctuate that even in love, where less is at stake, diagnosis is at the heart of decision making. Ultimately, however, this is probably the most tragic of the subplots, given that the nurse's diagnosis *is* malignant, and her lover will leave her because he can't imagine going to the beach with her, entering a party with her on his arm, having sex, undressing her, feeling her stump beneath him: "Look, Vivian. I've thought about it and you'll be better off."[25]

This novel uses diagnosis at every turn. Diagnosis creates a hierarchy of authority, an aura of suspense. The novel introduces the reader to the weighty power of diagnosis in the hospital and in the lives of the patients, the doctors, and the hospital administrators. As the nursing students learn about the power of diagnosis, the readers do by proxy, being instructed about the awe in which diagnosis should be held. After all, in *The Final Diagnosis*, it explains every success and every downfall.

Diagnostic revelations wend in and out of Serbian-American Téa Obreht's first novel, *The Tiger's Wife*, part of a story about survival in times of war and in the face of inevitable death.[26] One might be forgiven for thinking that the pivotal diagnostic moment is the hidden one, alluded to in the early pages of the book. Natalia, through whose voice the story is told, is a doctor and the granddaughter of an esteemed and recently deceased doctor whose soul's meanderings, as projected by Natalia, are the frame for this book. In the first chapter, she learns of her grandfather's unexpected death in a remote town that no one in her family has heard of before. He had announced to his wife that he was joining Natalia on a goodwill vaccination mission in a children's orphanage in the post-war Balkans. Natalia was not aware that he intended to join her and expected he was too sick to do so in any case. She does know he has cancer, a diagnosis which was disclosed to him in her presence, but which is kept secret between the two. To keep the diagnosis from his wife, he invents patients who he says he is going out to treat when in fact, he is going for his own treatment. We will learn no more about his diagnosis. However, diagnosis will shape the narrative nonetheless.

The location of the grandfather's death, far from home, is troublesome; in the Balkan culture in which this story is set, a soul has 40 days to revisit the places of its past before, hopefully, being called home by his familiar objects and loved ones. Natalia must locate the clinic to recover his personal effects and return them to her grandmother, to enhance the chances that her grandfather will find his way home. But at the same time, she also navigates the places of her grandfather's past, as might his soul. This journey is the foundation for the novel. By telling his story (and many other folk stories as well), Natalia is locating his soul as much as she is locating the physical possessions that she is tasked with returning to her grandmother. As Natalia visits his past, she will anchor its narrative between two other stories: "Everything necessary to understand my grandfather lies between two stories: the story of the tiger's wife, and the story of the deathless man"[27] she writes by way of introduction. The deathless man, as we soon find out, cannot die, much as he would like to. He has already been shot many times and has drowned. His accidents are incompatible with life, but

he lives on. In this section, I turn my attention to the story of the deathless man.

The deathless man is a doctor but also the nephew of Death. He
makes it his work to let people know they are going to die. But unlike
the grim reaper, he is not there simply to collect them; he visits them
before they die to name their disease. When he encounters Natalia's
grandfather, it is after having been killed (but not dying) at the hand
of a man whom he diagnosed: "He was dying of tuberculosis – you've
heard what they're saying around the village, I'm sure. I only came to
tell him, to help him, to be here when it happened. Come now, Doctor – blood on pillows, a terrible cough. What was your diagnosis even
before you came here?"[28]

The deathless man's and grandfather's paths cross several times
during the narrative, and at each encounter, their conversations will
revolve around the subjects of diagnosis and of death. The deathless
man distinguishes clearly between the two: "'People used to die from
death,' he explained. 'It's different today.'"[29]

The deathless man comes to realize over the course of the story,
which is bounded by the lifespan of the grandfather, that his greatest
gift is not in pronouncing the diagnosis to the person; rather it is in
indulging those who are going to die so that they needn't be destabi-
lized by the diagnosis of a fatal disease. "It is through that not-knowing
that [the person] will not suffer,"[30] he explains, making reference to the
tremendous transformative power of the diagnostic utterance that we
have discussed in the previous chapters. He does, however, stay nearby
to witness the death and to make things easier for his uncle by "round-
ing up [the newly deceased] and making sure they don't get lost during
their 40 days."

But diagnosis is not the sole preserve of the deathless man, or of
medicine, for that matter, in *The Tiger's Wife*. The apothecary, who it
turns out is an evil man, gains favour by diagnosis. He recognized
its powers, and was "a giver of answers, the vanquisher of fear, the
restorer of order and stability." He too presents the townspeople with
diagnoses; however, he is not medically trained. He comes up with
predictions that are frequently accurate and rides a tide of luck for
a very long time. He sees diagnosis as the access to the "real power"
that "lay in the definite and the concrete, in predictions backed by evidence, in the continued life of a man you claimed you could save, and
the death of a man you pronounced was certain to die."[31] While the
apothecary will use his power to kill, the deathless man is powerless

to change the outcome of his diagnoses, linked as they are to his uncle's indomitable reach.

This book uses diagnosis and the various doctors' tales to set out the stakes. It provides a means of oscillating between revelation and secret, certainty and oblivion, duty and destiny. But importantly, it underlines the way in which diagnosis variably contributes to, or detracts from, eternal salvation. Like the deathless man, Natalia is both a diagnostician and a rounder-up of souls. She makes the same journey as her grandfather's soul in her narrative, enabling her grandfather to return to the family for his eternal rest.

Diagnosis is everywhere in mainstream fiction. Not only does it serve important plot-shaping roles as I have described in the examples above, but it can also intercede in subtler ways in countless other works of fiction. In crime thrillers, diagnosis surfaces regularly. In Susan Hill's *The Various Haunts of Men*, for example, a character who is diagnosed with cancer uses her diagnosis to help the police.[32] She opts for alternative medicine to treat her malignant breast cancer but stays in close contact with her general practitioner (who is the triplet sister of the police chief) investigating a "psychic surgeon" who they believe may have been killing his patients. She arranges to see this psychic surgeon as a simultaneously factitious and real patient and contributes to his downfall and arrest. (In a later book in the series, we find out that her malignant disease has disappeared, along with her husband.)

In *Helsinki White*, it is the police officer who is diagnosed.[33] A national police hero, Inspector Kari Vaara has been suffering from blinding headaches, which it turns out are due to a brain tumour. After his (successful) surgery, he finds that he is no longer able to feel any emotion. That condition enables him to turn from good cop to bad, from public protector to psychopath.

But diagnosis can also be used as a kind of background decoration, with a less pivotal role than those in the crime thrillers. One of my favourite scenes discussing diagnostic disclosure (after *Saturday*, that is) is in an entertaining book by Simon Kemelman, *Wednesday the Rabbi Got Wet*.[34] This series, with one book for each day of the week, highlights the tribulations of a Boston North Shore Conservative Jewish community whose awkward intellectual rabbi uses Talmudic reasoning and pilpul (a form of scholarly argument) to assist his good friend, an Irish American police chief, to resolve numerous crimes.

A prominent member of the community dies from an allergy to a prescribed antibiotic. While figuring out whether the doctor mis-prescribed or the pharmacists incorrectly filled the order, or some other devious intervention took place, a discussion and characterization of the doctor takes place. Their discussion, not unlike the one I highlighted in the Introduction underlines the degree to which the way a doctor delivers a diagnosis, what affect a doctor assumes, matters in the construction of the profession. To give the readers a sense of what the doctor in question (Dr Daniel Cohen) is like, the readers overhear a discussion about him between two of his colleagues. One of them explains:

> You take the average patient ... he needs assurance that his doctor knows just what's wrong with him and just what will cure him ... What I'm saying is, your patient has to look up to you. With Dan Cohen, he's like your uncle who tells you to rub yourself with chicken fat to cure your arthritis. See what I mean? ... Dan is like the old-fashioned family-type doctor, the kind that used to sit up half the night with a pneumonia patient waiting for the crisis. Well, that attitude is out nowadays. People are suspicious. They think if you're too anxious, you must have some sort of angle, like maybe you don't know what's wrong and you don't want to admit it. Or maybe you made the wrong diagnosis and gave the wrong medication.[35]

Diagnosis also features widely in stories about love, using the delivery of a serious diagnosis to put into stark contrast the urgency and the simultaneous banality of life. Hearing a lover's diagnosis identifies a potentially newly limited term to a relationship one imagined (or at least hoped) was unlimited. The diagnosis of a spouse gives an opportunity for the narrator or protagonist in a work of fiction to tussle with the idea of his or her own mortality through the diagnosis offered to their other half. While we know our lives and those of our loved ones *will* end, we do not usually have a clear sense of how that end will occur. The diagnostic moment, when it's a dire prognosis, brings that mortality into harsh reality.

In *Vital Signs*, the narrator grapples with his contesting emotions of both love and hate for his wife of 30 years when he learns of her diagnosis.[36] The story starts not at the onset of symptoms but at the final diagnostic workup, each step in the build-up to the final verdict further plunging him into turmoil: "I am not worthy," he writes. Anna's diagnosis may mean he may never be able to cleanse himself by admitting a past infidelity

On the other hand, in *Gilead*, the fictional narrator is coming to terms with his own diagnosis and its impact on relationships with his loved ones.[37] A minister, he writes this epistolary novel to his very young son, tracing the family and social history, while propounding lessons for his son if he is not there to teach him in person, the lessons at the same time pastoral and paternal. So too is his account of his own diagnosis: "The doctor used the term *'angina pectoris,'* which has a theological sound, like *Misericordia*," he explains. "I can only be grateful. I do regret that I have almost nothing to leave you and your mother."[38]

In *Complicity*, I didn't expect the diagnosis that arrived in the last pages of the novel.[39] There had been clues, but I had either ignored them, or not seen them for what they were. In this crime thriller, a journalist, Cameron Colley, is clearly being set up for a series of almost unreadably horrific murders of high-profile, successful men. The story is told in a broken narrative with three different threads. The continuous narrative is the first-person account by the journalist in relation to the murders. It is interspersed with stories from his past, which initially seem to be explaining his own behaviours to the reader, when, in fact, they are (as we find out) revealing information about the murderer. The third narrative, written in second person, is from the murderer himself whose identity is not made clear until the end, just before Colley's diagnosis. In this classic noir thriller, as the plot moves towards resolution, the cough that Colley has been nursing throughout the book (this reader, for one, thought the cough served simply to underline Colley's couldn't-care-less, hard-smoking character), turns out to be lung cancer. As the killer's identity is revealed, so is Colley's malignant diagnosis. The Colley narration, post-diagnosis, shifts to the second person, punctuating, in true noir style, his simultaneous role as victim and as transgressor, not unlike that of the murderer.

Diagnosis plays so many important social roles as it infiltrates these fictional accounts. I do not want, for a moment, to suggest that these diagnostic scenes represent reality, should represent reality, or serve as models in any way of what diagnosis is (or should be). On the other hand, what they demonstrate with aplomb is the manner in which diagnosis can be used symbolically in a work of literary fiction. As we consider these symbolic uses, we may also be able to glean a deeper sense of what diagnosis can come to represent in our conceptualization of health, illness, and disease, rightly or wrongly.

I stop for a moment to refer to Eviatar Zerubavel's sociological work. This is not because he writes about diagnosis (he doesn't). However, he postulates that the work of the social scholar is to consider not just empirical, observable, controlled instances of particular social occurrences. Rather, it is to look more widely at social phenomena in all their manifestations and forms. Can we see evidence of a social pattern, that is to say, an example of the phenomena that transcends eras, media, and settings?[40] Can we speak, generally in this case, about what diagnosis tends to punctuate and how it conveys information about far more than disease in the settings in which it is used?

Fiction is a useful setting in which to observe diagnosis, diagnostic disclosure, and its social forms. Its usefulness is linked to the amazing and creative ways in which diagnosis can be put to use. For example, if we are to start with *Saturday*, as I did with the introduction to this chapter, the diagnostic scene was an important way of wresting control away from the thugs and throwing the *déroulement* of the event back into the expected social order, returning to the neurosurgeon the authority of his position. Of course, this control is short-lived, as Baxter will find Perowne in his home and try to regain his lost dignity with further assaults on Perowne and his family.

But Perowne will get the upper hand back, a second time. Just as with the deathless man, whose power emanated from supernatural sources, diagnosis punctuates social order and places all people at its mercy. Baxter can neither escape his disease, nor its label, and Perowne controls what it means.

In these depictions, diagnosis emanates from above, as part of the mystery of life, but it is delivered, explained, and palliated by particular agents of, variably, death (in the case of *The Tiger's Wife*) or medicine. There is a kind of natural order which is confirmed by the power to diagnose. This is an order that Dr Dan Cohen challenges (a bit) by his unconventional affect in *Wednesday the Rabbi Got Wet*.[41] He doesn't showcase his authority, appearing to his critics rather more like an old uncle than a modern-day doctor. However, he does not challenge it completely, because, as the readers discover, he is correct in his diagnosis and prescription, and being a nice guy hasn't actually interfered with his important diagnostic ability. However, the trials he has experienced and the suspicion to which he has been subject during the investigation (mainly by the laypeople in the congregation) underline that to diagnose and to be an agent of medicine is to be powerful in conventional sorts of ways and to assume a particular (epistemic) posture.

Another kind of power is exercised and distributed in these various fictitious renderings of diagnosis, in this case, handing some vestige of control back to the lay protagonists who have received a diagnosis. Lucy, in *The Final Diagnosis*, now an amputee, orders her boyfriend to consider whether he wants to spend his life with her. He does not actually leave her without her prodding, which, while devastating, leaves her in control of her future, despite the lack of control she may otherwise feel. Ruth, in *All That I Am*, similarly, finally is able to gain access to her repressed memories, and now has the ability (power) to commemorate greatness. Without her diagnosis, she would not be able to go back to the past, which alone can bring her cousin's greatness to the fore. In a sense, her diagnosis saves both her and her cousin.

In the same manner, Susan Hill's cancer victim can reveal the criminal and put an end to his murderous activities. At the same time, she will get better, against all logic, in the next book of the series. The Hill series bears mentioning because of the close relationship between the law and the diagnosis. Hill's main characters, Simon Serailler and his triplet sister Cat Deerborn are, respectively, police inspector and doctor. Both professions provide a kind of moral order, both constitute pursuit of the truth, of right and of wrong, of crime and of criminal. Both of the protagonists must engage in careful sleuthing, the art and intuition of the diagnostician, the consequences entailed by arriving upon the correct diagnosis, and indeed, the authority and prestige conveyed by the power to diagnose.

Complicity is the most recent of the books I describe here, not in terms of its publication, but in terms of when I read it. I found it just as I was finishing this chapter, a kind of hidden treasure: a book already on one of my shelves but that I hadn't yet read. As I said in the introduction to this chapter, I love the kind of book this one was clearly going to be: quickly paced with an intricate plot. But when I got to the last chapter, and all the murders were resolved, I stumbled across the diagnosis I described above:

> They say it's about the size of a tennis ball. You slide your hand inside your coat and jacket and press up under the floating rib on your left side.

Pain. You're not sure whether you can feel it, the thing, the growth itself or not; you cough a bit as you press, and the pain gets worse. You stop pressing and the pain eases.[42]

This unexpected turn – even with its precursor signs that I hadn't picked up on – changed the way I understood the whole book. Colley's innocence was barely gained when it was stolen, mirroring the loss of innocence as a teenager of his murdering friend. It further linked the two men, in an unexpected way.

But beyond that, I couldn't look past the parallels between the fictional diagnostic revelation and the very public revelation, some 20 years later, of the author's own terminal diagnosis. On 3 April 2013, Iain Banks wrote on his web page "I am officially Very Poorly." He explained that he had just received a diagnosis of gall bladder cancer, that it had spread, and that he would be retiring from public life. He told his fans that he had asked his partner if she would do him the honour "of becoming [his] widow" and then left on a honeymoon.[43] He died two and a half months later.

In Banks's personal statement, as in his novel, the diagnostic moment was what Art Frank would refer to as an epiphany. Following Denzin, Frank maintains that an epiphany is a moment of crisis that makes a mark on a person and reveals who they really are. He adds that for these moments of crisis to be able to make their mark on the individual, there has to be a "cultural milieu in which such experiences are at least possibilities, if not routine expectations."[44]

In one sense, Colley's diagnosis in *Complicity* (as in the innumerable other examples of diagnosis fiction) enabled Banks's personal epiphany. Diagnosis novels, plays, poems, and all of its other cultural forms give us the launching pad from which we can imagine our own diagnoses. We write them, we read them, and perhaps one day, we will experience them.

An earlier version of this chapter previously appeared in *Perspectives in Biology and Medicine*, volume 59, number 3 (summer 2016): 400–413. © 2017 by Johns Hopkins University Press.

CHAPTER FIVE

Breaking Bad:
The Diagnostic Moment in
Film and Television

with Thierry Jutel

Just as the diagnostic moment figures prominently in fiction, it also has a strong tradition in film and television. Yet stories told about diagnosis in these visual media have other ways for directing the viewer's attention and perspective than do written texts. Imagine the close-up of the character's face, the way in which the camera captures pain, joy, or concentration. Think how the music weaves between the images, using sombre tones, minor chords, or cacophony to punctuate pivotal action in the development of the narrative. Consider what it means for a character to cough. Is it a clue about what is going to happen?

Many of the narrative techniques in film and television are not available to the novelist or poet, and they make the stories of diagnosis very powerful on the screen in a different way. Similar to fiction, however, the diagnosis is a prevalent device, and pervades modern film and television, especially in relation to middle-class, white and usually, educated characters. The diagnoses in these films create highly personalized and emotionalized storylines, which then create an inside perspective on major social and cultural institutions, their forms of knowledge, and power.

The diagnosis scene is, of course, ubiquitous in the hospital drama (*Grey's Anatomy*, *The Good Doctor*, *Code Black*) where the dramatic tensions tend to focus on the subjective, emotional, and psychological traits of medical professionals and patients. It was even the topic of at least one television series. *House, MD*, like Hailey's *The Final Diagnosis*, used diagnosis as a central theme to underscore the tensions present in the institutional context of a hospital, medical hierarchies, and the relation between expertise and power with the human foibles of its central character. It was the pretext for the show, and even though Dr House's diagnostic prowess doesn't quite redeem him as a character in the eyes of his viewers the way it does Dr Pearson in *The Final Diagnosis* (House is terribly flawed if not unlikeable), it redeems his actions and explains his devoted following. In *House,* diagnostic discovery is the outcome of deduction, of forensic acumen. House's ability to connect observations and evidence systematically and intuitively is the result of his intellectual and deductive skills. But genius has a price; the talented and mercurial diagnostician is himself in need of diagnostic assessment. Is he a rebel or a pathfinder within the medical establishment, an addict, a psychopath, a melancholic?

Diagnostic revelations in films also occur when they are least expected and in films that are not about medicine. There are diagnoses in popular TV series (*Breaking Bad,* of course; *Sopranos*; and even *Madmen*), in French art house films (*Repas de Noël, Same old Song*), and in major Hollywood films (*Still Alice, Side Effects*).

The ways in which diagnosis serves as a trigger for filmic and televisual stories are similar but not identical to the narratives we see in diagnosis fiction. In many ways, it's more explicit than in novels. Films such as *Still Alice* and *Iris* have diagnosis as their premise. We go into the cinema expecting the diagnosis, even knowing ahead of the characters who will be diagnosed what will happen to them. But, even when diagnosis is not the focus of the film, it may still be its most important framing device. The diagnosis may launch the film, or appear in the early part of the story, setting the scene for what follows. Or it may come very late in the film, as a surprise, and be used as an explanatory device for some other conundrum.

Diagnosis is a useful tool in the scriptwriter's bag as it captures and synthesizes the life of characters and establishes their predicament very quickly. It generates drama instantly and captures the attention of the viewer; it locates stories within the context of the medical institution, which is central to a contemporary Western understanding of the social; and it plays with our emotional allegiances and our capacity for understanding and compassion. The representation of the diagnostic moment and connected moments of power and medical and health institutions, social relations, and emotional impact provide the ingredients to reproduce, question, or explore health, life, and death. It also addresses some of the key ingredients of narrative such as causality and the modalities of change through which characterization can be explored and enhanced,[1] as it traces the journey of characters when diagnostic announcement and revelation occur function as key turning points.[2] Diagnosis is a profoundly social moment that provides powerful potential for narrative purposes in these visual media. In contemporary Western, middle-class cultures, where characters rely on their social status for recognition and entitlement, the announcement of a serious illness provides a powerful form of destabilization.

The number of films that rely upon diagnosis as a prominent narrative device is impressive. There are so many we can't write about them all. However, we will describe a few of them here and show how they contribute to the way in which we imagine the diagnostic moment. We have chosen a mix of films and TV dramas that typify some of the uses that are made of diagnostic revelation.

Not only are the techniques of narrative that uses a diagnosis different in film and television from the diagnostic revelation used in written fiction, but there are also structural differences. Most narrative films, and certainly Hollywood cinema, are driven by cause-and-effect structures that impact characters and whose trajectory, transformations, and ways of dealing with circumstances provide the fictional interest and means through which spectators invest in the story.[3] Diagnostic moments – turning points in the lives of characters – provide ready-made plot elements around which the narrative can be launched or altered and the characters revealed to themselves and to viewers. Since most narrative cinema is structured around what script writers label "inciting incidents," diagnosis becomes a handy tool. A character is defined or redefined in the dramatic revelation of an illness that now either has or does not have a name and requires the character to understand, respond, and digest the moment. The diagnosis is an inciting incident par excellence.

For the viewer, the disclosure of a diagnosis – and especially in the case of a high-profile disease (say, cancer, Alzheimer's, or Zika) – is an intense moment in which the tools of visual storytelling can be mobilized (close-up; shot-reverse-shot editing, music and silence) and, as we will see below, to the point of becoming abstract and stylized televisual and cinematic moments. It also enables the production of a motivated narrative structure based on the revelation of character through reaction. Viewers do not simply follow the characters' actions in the moment and the aftershock of diagnostic announcement but also contemplate how they themselves process the information. Since, as Bordwell argues, characters are revealed by action, the reaction of the character contributes an important ingredient to the storytelling.[4] Everything in the character's reaction will take on meaning, even if it is only an unfocused stare, or a distracted response such as when Walter White, in *Breaking Bad*, fixates on his doctor's food-stained lab coat,[5] a scene replicated in the French film *Médecin de campagne*.[6]

The diagnostic scene with the food-stained lab coat in *Breaking Bad*,[7] which takes place in the first episode of the series, provides a particularly salient example. Walter White's discovery of his terminal cancer launches events that reveal and transform him in radical and surprising ways. The prologue to the series shows Walter White, high school chemistry teacher and part-time car wash attendant, barrelling down a desert road in a recreational vehicle and recording what sounds like a last letter to his family. This puzzling and unexplained series of events is followed by the credit sequence and then a day in the insipid life of Walter White on his 50th birthday in which his social standing and masculinity are challenged.

The day starts with Walter exercising early in the morning on a ridiculously small exercise device (a "mini stepper") when he starts coughing. While coughing is a rather innocuous occurrence in real life, in cinema and television it is always a portent of something sombre. The day unfolds with Walter being served vegan bacon instead of the real thing for breakfast as a "treat," teaching chemistry to bored and belligerent high school students, going to his second job in a car wash service shop where some his students see him wash cars and mock him, and finally returning to a surprise birthday party. While he is supposed to be the centre of attention, his brother-in-law, a drug enforcement agent, steals the show with tales of drug arrests and the display of his impressive handgun. Later in the evening, his wife masturbates him while she follows on her laptop the final throes of online bidding for an object she has put on sale. When the bidding is finally over and she sells the object above the set reserve, she explodes with joy while Walter remains puzzled and sexually unsatisfied but mostly demeaned. This series of events implying his impotence, culminates literally and metaphorically the next day when, working at the car wash, he collapses in a fit of coughing and is transported to the emergency room by ambulance.

The diagnostic sequence (figure 5.1) follows shortly after his ambulance trip with a high angle shot right above Walter as he glides into the MRI machine with its loud and distracting whirring sounds. His

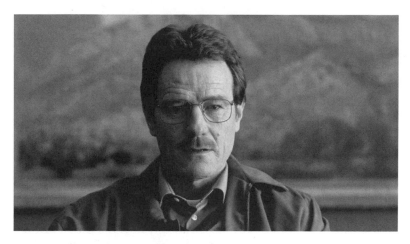

5.1 Walter White (Brian Cranston) receiving the diagnosis
of inoperable lung cancer, in *Breaking Bad*.

head is upside down, his eyes moving side to side. The next shot offers a graphic match as it features a reflection of Walter's face on the
physician's varnished desk. A tilting movement of the camera then
reframes the shot with Walter's passive and puzzled expression now
prominently displayed. Walter focuses first on the doctor's lips, shown
in slow motion, and then on a spot of mustard on the doctor's lab coat
lapel. The physician is speaking but the sound is at first an expression-
istic mix of buzzing sounds and inaudible words until the doctor's
voice becomes audible:

"Mr White?" We hear the clear voice of the doctor interceding. "Mr
White?"
  "Yes?"
  "You've understood what I've just said to you?"
  "Yes. Lung cancer. Inoperable."
  "I'm sorry. I just need to make sure you fully understand."
  "Best case scenario, with chemo, I'll live maybe another couple a
years ... It's just ... you've got mustard on your ... right there ... mus-
tard ... there ... right there [pointing]."

He says it and for the first time has a smug expression of content-
ment, as if the comment about the mustard stain could diffuse the

significance of the diagnosis and the prognosis and give him a measure
of advantage over the purveyor of bad news.

While the sequence is short and lacks a kind of narrative digestion
of its dramatic implications, the significance of the moment is most
obviously captured in the highly stylized aural and visual treatment
of the sequence: acute camera angles, distorted sounds, slow motion,
shallow then deep focus cinematography, and a composition that emphasizes stasis and distance combine to produce an unemotional and
depersonalized feel to the moment. The diagnostic scene leaves us with
a feeling of unreality and uncertainty (how is the protagonist taking
the news?) as if the impact of the news is going to be revealed in other
moments of the episode. This is a pattern we will see in most of the examples we discuss: the clinician's diagnostic announcement is rarely a
sequence where the patient/protagonist fully absorbs the implications
of the news. Indeed, the hectic prologue that opens in the middle of
what seems like a chase and a moment in which Walter White contem-
plates his mortality (he does leave a recorded message to his family) is,
because of the art of narrative construction and the viewer's search for
coherent meaning, the rejoinder to the passivity of Walter White in the
clinician's office. How does the absent-minded and impotent Walter
White end up in the desert wearing only underwear, a shirt, and a gas
mask and in a moment of utter panic?

What we come to realize in the first episode of the series is that
this conventional (albeit repressed and emasculated) family man and
teacher will, via this diagnosis, metamorphose into a different person.
Depending on how you read this he either throws off his chains and
realizes his real self, or he becomes a new someone else. In any case, he
will recruit an errant student to help him manufacture methamphet-
amine to finance his treatment and secure his family's future once he
dies. He will break the law, become a drug lord, kill people, and assume
a completely different set of values and behaviours while keeping the
pretense of being the same person but afflicted by an incurable disease.
He will become the opposite of Walter White, assuming the alternative
persona of "Heisenberg," a cold-blooded and calculating criminal who
will become a terrifying figure and an urban legend, and ultimately a
source of existential enjoyment and a death-wish for Walter. "Chemistry is the study of change," declares Walter in his science classroom: the
premise of the television series is to trace the most radical of individual
transformations and for the viewer to make sense of this anti-hero's
journey.

Diagnosis in *Breaking Bad* is the study of discarding social norms under the pretext of urgency and existential duty. Diagnosis and prognosis in *Breaking Bad* are not sentences but liberation: the television series plays with our desire to see characters change, learn, and overcome. "Growth, then decay, then transformation" Walter pronounces in the same science lesson: the premise of the show is to cast his white, middle-aged, and frustrated character into a set of circumstances in which his response to illness is to transgress social norms, paradoxically in the name of family. As other commentators have mentioned, the series invites an allegorical interpretation about the state of lower-middle-class white masculinity.[8] In other words, the medical diagnosis is itself the premise for a societal and political diagnosis. Diagnosis in the examples we discuss here always gives rise to narrative of social connections and dislocations.

While film deploys, as described above, the tools of cinematic storytelling to produce dramatic structure, motivation, character traits, and narrative causality, it also puts generic conventions at work. Genre, is the way in which a text (in this case, a visual text, but it applies to all texts and all forms of communication) creates "effects of reality and truth, authority and plausibility, which are central to the different ways in which the world is understood."[9] While an individual film always functions as structure of signification and emotion unto itself, it is always also positioned in relation to broader contexts, such as genre.

The rules of genres are familiar to both film-makers and audiences, and provide ways for constructing character and emotion. Genre relies on the fact that the audience will be able to recognize narrative and cinematic components, such as stock characters, situations, styles, or even shots. It is always, as Frow describes in his book on genre, revealing new information on the basis of old information in a compressed form. This includes, for example, the voice-over narration in film noir, the absence of the reverse shot in the horror film, and the introduction of music to demarcate narrative, emotional, and psychological excess in the melodrama. Narratives are always at work in each individual film and in the compulsory nature of generic repetition.

Diagnostic moments provide an especially acute example of this articulation of singular occurrence and known event. The announcement of a diagnosis is both a moment of suspension (the world is reorganized around the character whose life is now transformed) and a familiar event that the cues of genre help viewers to recognize. Some of these cues will be delivered through the conventions of melodrama, which Peter Brooks describes as less of a literary genre and as more of a mode,[10] and which Thomas Elsaesser extended to cinema and the family melodrama.[11] These cues include the themes of fate and the individual in an alienating social world where emotions and aspirations can never be channelled into redeeming social acts or contained within the forces of ideological repression.[12]

One genre that makes significant use of diagnostic moments is melodrama, which always reveals a discrepancy between the experience of grief and disempowerment and the social means to express those. The films we discuss below work with and around some of the melodramatic conventions of cinema to negotiate what we have described as the inherent tension of the diagnostic scene, where the naming of a disease introduces important narrative functions.

Many films use the diagnostic revelation as a means of underscoring acceptance and sacrifice, for example, *Iris*,[13] *Love Story*,[14] and *I've Loved You So Long*.[15] We have chosen *Still Alice* as an exemplar.[16] This 2014 film, starring Julianne Moore and Alec Baldwin, depicts a successful 50-something female professor of linguistics who learns that she has early-onset Alzheimer's disease. *Still Alice* illustrates what appears to be the dominant narrative use of diagnosis: the character's ability to assume the diagnosis and its transformative power. Because of the nature of her diagnosis, her children are also advised to have genetic screening and the results predict that one of her daughters is also at risk. The diagnosis reorganizes the relations within the family, as Alice both is the centre of attention (she is the sick person) and loses all self-agency as a result of the diagnosis, despite her efforts to organize her future, including preparing instructions for herself on how to end her life. In melodramatic terms, this can be cast as the transcending nature of the experience and the possibility of illness as self-sacrifice which reveals the strength and determination of a character whose selflessness emphasizes her devotion and courage. In other words, *Still Alice* is centrally concerned with suffering and virtue.

The narrative progresses along the expected pathway of her disease by capturing Alice's responses to new challenges brought about by her progressive impairment, her loss of herself, and her family's management of the circumstances. The narrative is, apart from the initial diagnostic moment, structured around events that imply chronological continuity and Alice's progressive disappearance (both metaphorically and literally) and increasingly subtle touches of self-awareness and agency the character demonstrates. It also reveals characters and especially those connected to the family and the domestic sphere.

Alice's experience of illness is, in melodramatic tradition, highly gendered. Her progressive departure from herself emphasizes a particular grace and serenity linked to femininity. This points to the possibility of closure in terms of narrative (she withdraws gracefully) and the insistence of her humanity over the power of her disease, despite the fact that her professional, personal, and domestic lives have collapsed.

The emphasis of traditionally feminine roles such as mother, wife, and professionals facing gender-based injustices is common to melodrama (often grouped in a sub-genre called "women's films"[17]). In these films, the dramatic events in the female character's social and personal life reveal inextricable circumstances that the female character is forced to accept. The emotional and narrative premise is not so much the overcoming of forces of repression of the female character but her resilience. In *Still Alice*, Alice becomes closer to a daughter from whom she had grown distant, but inversely her husband leaves her for a job he thinks he cannot refuse; their respective life trajectories move apart. He disappears from her life and the narrative and the wrongs he has committed are left without explanation, justification, or resolution.

The film follows Alice's emotional journey as character and underplays the broader social, medical, financial, and institutional context of her illness. The fact that the character is introduced early on as a successful academic in an upper-middle-class setting justifies this ellipsis but also allows for the contrasting images of a self-reliant woman and a person in need of constant care. In this, and in other films (see *The Decline of the American Empire*,[18] for example, and the other films discussed in this chapter), the protagonist is an educated and articulate person who has the material and emotional resources to rationalize and understand their illness and express emotions. He or she projects a sense of entitlement that is dramatically challenged by the unpredictable and unmanageable arrival of the illness and its confirmation in the highly ritualized diagnostic announcement.

The means of telling the story do not solely rely on the social and psychological traits of the character; because cinematic means contribute to showing the progression of Alice's disease via the shifting significance of the visual motif of Alice shot on her own, even when she is with other people. This includes the opening shot of the film, which rather than providing an establishing shot of the family around a restaurant table as they celebrate her birthday, focuses exclusively on Alice even though the first voice we hear is her daughter's ("Okay. Happy birth-day, Mom"). This type of shot constitutes a visual motif that allows the viewer to trace the progression of the narrative through Alice's per-spective and response, and helps measure the shifting signification of her disease.

This invitation to the viewer to measure the shifting mental state of Alice is, in traditionally narrative terms, foreshadowed in the first sequence where Alice inappropriately responds to her daughter's mention of sibling rivalry by referring to her own youth. The implied temporal dislocation initiates the narrative and the viewer's recogni-tion of symptoms from the start. Viewers will already be aware of the premise of the narrative, the story of a woman who struggles with the realities of early-onset Alzheimer's. The diagnostic announcement is therefore not a source of suspense, but the emerging symptoms of her illness focus the viewer's attention and generate a form of diagnostic deciphering and a compassionate response to Alice's predicament: she is, in traditional standards of contemporary Western society, an accom-plished, strong, independent, and successful woman. In other words, the motif of Alice captured in visual isolation marks the progression of the narrative, the emergence of Alice's confusion, and the dramatic implication of the disease, and provides the means for the viewer to observe Alice's reaction.

The scenes relating to the diagnostic process, from Alice's entry into a medical context to the sharing of the diagnostic pronouncements with close family members, take place early in the narrative. There are five of them, all interrelated: the first is Alice's appointment with a neuro-psychiatrist where she reveals her symptoms and worries that she has a brain tumour. The physician suggests some diagnostic tests, in par-ticular, an MRI. The second occurs when Alice returns to the neuropsy-chiatrist and he tells her that she might have Alzheimer's disease. The third occurs when Alice tells her husband. The fourth takes place when the neuropsychiatrist confirms the diagnosis to Alice and her husband, and the final happens when Alice and her husband announce her diag-nosis to the children and recommend they be tested. The five sequences function as necessary moments in the narrative progression. Each one involves a combination of different characters and focuses on different aspects of Alice's experiences.

In the first diagnostic sequence, the scene starts with a sound-bridge transition: after a run during which Alice got lost on her campus and returns home, obviously distressed, her voice is heard off-screen providing an account of the pattern she has observed about her mental lapses. The images in the viewers' mind of Alice in total panic at home contrasted with her detached telling of what she was experiencing ("I started to forget things, little annoying things like words and names. And I got lost, completely lost running on campus") emphasize the intense gap between her disorienting experience of symptoms and her capacity to rationally and calmly describe these experiences.

As the next shot reveals Alice in a brightly lit and quite bland space in shallow focus (we see very little beyond Alice's face), another voice breaks in and immediately positions this interlocutor as a medical specialist quizzing Alice about her general health and any other possible explanations. The still-yet-to-be-seen-in-shot male doctor asks Alice to memorize a random name and address that he will ask her (and indirectly the viewer) to recall later on. The dialogue is now clearly part of a diagnostic process where Alice's confident, clear, and slightly puzzled account is translated into diagnostic clues. The conversation shifts to a series of simple questions ("What's your name?" "What day is it?") all of them Alice answers with confidence and an expression and tone of slight amusement. She answers questions about her family and medical history. She mentions the dramatic death of her mother and a sibling in a car accident when she was young and the death of her father from what she described as his alcoholism and cirrhosis.

Predictably, as the neuropsychiatrist asks her to recall the name and address he gave her shortly before, Alice struggles to remember even after he gives clues. For the first time, she becomes defensive; she dismisses, rationalizes, relativizes, and explains her incapacity to remember the information he gave her. She worries aloud that she has a brain tumour, which is less an explanation of her symptoms and more evidence that she is so perturbed by her health that she has diagnosed herself and has focused her anxiety on an illness that would fit her age and her understanding and possibly experience of what might cause such dysfunction. While the physician makes no pronouncements, he recommends further tests. For the viewer, there is no suspense about the cause of her symptoms but rather empathy for Alice's denial. That compassion is highlighted by the fact that even for the viewer, it's hard to remember the address, and this engages the viewer with Alice's anxiety.

Throughout this entire sequence, the camera's focus remains on a single and motionless shot of Alice's face in a medium close-up, without a single cut and for a remarkable three minutes. This is a long take without any camera movements and with no significant actions except for Alice's expressions and reactions. This is remarkable in terms of the conventions of contemporary mainstream cinema as such a shot calls attention to itself. The medical doctor is off-screen, not seen in the sequence; the camera is singularly focused on Alice, a pattern relating to the visual motif of her isolation in the shots noted above. The scene, in screenwriting terminology, is *an inciting incident*, which becomes the turning point after which her life cannot be the same, a moment of transformative power. In narrative terms, the symptoms and her display of anxiety ineluctably leads to the dramatic revelation of her fate. In this instance and in many other films with diagnostic announcements, the revelation and acknowledgment of symptoms has an instrumentalized function in the narrative. It advances the story and challenges the character whose evolution and transformation audiences will observe and measure and with which they will be affectively and emotionally connected. And to emphasize the dramatic turn in the narrative and the sudden threat to Alice's fate, the subsequent shot is an exterior one with tree branches covered with ice, shot in shallow depth of field, which renders most of the shot blurry: only the tip of that branch is in focus.

In the next sequence we see the family Christmas dinner where Alice is the focus of our attention and where she shows an increased degree of self-monitoring (she tests her memory while preparing Christmas dinner). At the close of the sequence, she unambiguously demonstrates to the viewer, but not to herself, that her memory is failing badly. The viewer is given the privileged position of knowing before Alice what she is about to learn.

The second moment scene is when she returns to the doctor. There is some similarity in the sequence: the first shot is a medium close-up of Alice's face as he rules out, off-screen, a number of potential diagnoses, including the brain tumour that Alice had suggested as a cause of her symptoms. He also shares for the first time, his diagnostic hypothesis. At this point, and for the first time in the film, there is a cut to the doctor in medium close-up as he pronounces, "You have sporadic memory impairment, totally out of proportion to your age, and there is evidence of decline in your level of mental function." He suggests that Alzheimer's disease is a likely explanation for her symptoms: "You do fit the criteria." The prospective diagnosis emphasizes the empirically based relation between the observations and grouping of symptoms, the medical evidence of the disease, and the uncontested acceptance of medical authority, a point cinematically stressed by the first visual appearance of the physician as he makes the first pronouncement about her "impairment."

While he describes the potential explanation for her symptoms, the camera focuses on Alice's response. She has come to her appointment alone, despite his request she bring a family member, and there is no room for her to externalize her emotions. At the same time, there is no suspense: the viewer knows what is coming.

The mise en scène of this sequence, including setting and performance, as well as the editing, emphasize the institutionalized interaction: the roles and functions of patient and physician are implied and the process of diagnosis is bypassed to focus on the uncontested delivery of a medical mode of interpretation of symptoms as fact. The film treats this sequence economically in the sense that none of the impact of the information lands fully in the character or in the emotional emphasis in the film, even though viewers will have already noted memory slippages and disorientation but have not yet been given space and time to register the impact on the character.

The first emotional pay-off of Alice's realization of her condition comes in the third diagnostic sequence immediately following her visit to the specialist. Early in the morning after a sleepless night when, she rouses her husband and reveals her potential diagnosis: "They think it might be early-onset Alzheimer's disease." Instead of the slightly bemused and highly rational account of her symptoms we saw in her doctor's appointment, and in the face of her husband's surprise and denial ("This is insane!"), she confesses she is scared and reels off a list of symptoms.

Her husband, himself a medical researcher, seeks to reassure her by making a statement that is both declarative and questioning: "but there is no diagnosis yet (?)" Alice protests: "Damn it. Why would you not take me seriously? No, I know what I'm feeling. I know what it's feeling. It feels like my brain is fucking dying and everything I've worked for in my entire life is going!" She finally breaks down and sobs in his arms. This moment reveals their relationship as intimate and serene and in the subsequent breakfast scene ("Whatever happens, I'm here"), yet will be transformed into distance and alienation as the narrative advances.

The fourth diagnostic scene occurs when the actual diagnosis is revealed. The scene is anti-climactic in the sense that it is devoid of emotion but adds a narrative twist. The doctor's expertise and authority take precedence over Alice's ownership of her symptoms even if she did not have an explanatory narrative to make sense of them. The physician is the first to speak in this sequence as he presents the irrefutable evidence of the disease even when Alice's husband queries the conclusions he has drawn. In this interchange between physician and husband, a contest of medical practitioners unfolds; there is no room for Alice's own reaction. The scene concludes not with Alice's reaction to the diagnostic announcement but with the revelation that her illness could be genetic – that her children too, might develop the disease.

The fifth scene in which the diagnostic announcement is fully shaped as a social, personal, and emotional moment is key in terms of the overall narrative. Alice tells her two daughters (one of whom is married and pregnant and whose husband is present) and son that she has early-onset Alzheimer's disease. The sequence plays itself out beyond the medical and practical detachment of the earlier diagnostic moments: the fabric of the family and the ties between each member are instantly revealed in the ways they react and interact with one another. The scene is the emotional and social climax of the inciting incident we referred to above. That the disease can be transmitted across generations is a key ingredient driving the narrative. In contrast to Alice's own response, her children experience the gamut of attitudes from fear and denial to incomprehension and compassion.

The disclosure of the diagnosis is the starting point for a narrative exploration of illness as a familial and social trajectory, a dramatic event to be managed and controlled and yet revealed to others. The family sequence demonstrates Alice's increasing isolation, while later in the film she will grow closer to her previously distant and even estranged daughter to form, in melodramatic tradition, the terms of a resilient form of female bonding. Her visual depiction as alone in the shot shifts from that of an assured, successful, and empowered woman, to that of a lonely figure. In the last shots of the sequence, she is isolated. Her husband, earlier shown sitting next to her, is no longer in shot. She is transformed into a sick person in other people's eyes. Family members start talking about her as if she were not there, using the third person. The diagnostic revelation in the medical context paradoxically did not inscribe her narratively as transformed; it is her family's response that changes her from a driven and self-reliable character to a person whose existence is now entirely shaped by others' knowledge and discourse about her illness.

As if this were the revelation that mattered most to Alice, at the end of that sequence she finally breaks down. Music arises in the background (a rare occurrence in the film's emotional moments), and she asks her children for forgiveness. The sequence is over, and viewers do not see the reactions of the family members.

This scene completes the impact of the diagnosis pronouncement in its narrative trajectory. It also drives the rest of the film as Alice's illness and the family's reaction to her illness paradoxically reveals Alice's determination and the character of each family member. Her husband lets her down by accepting a new job that sees him move away when it is clearly not in Alice's best interest, and the wayward daughter becomes Alice's carer. In this sense, the diagnosis ends up "diagnosing" the other characters in the film. Following melodramatic conventions, Alice's fate provides the terms by which her immediate world is organized and where those who are close to her find and occupy roles, including through their metaphorical and actual disappearance from the film. The rest of the film traces Alice's decline and social erasure. The meaning of the title becomes clear as it evokes Alice's double journey as she becomes socially, physically, and emotionally still while struggling to remain herself. The significant narrative events in the film trace this progression and the oscillation in the stilling of Alice.

A Late Quartet[19] explores the impact of the life-altering diagnosis of Parkinson's disease on Peter Mitchell (played by Christopher Walken), the cellist in, and oldest member of, a world-renowned string quartet, and the implication that this long-standing musical partnership will come to an end. While this film, like *Still Alice*, is also a melodrama, that the diagnosed character is male changes the place that the diagnostic revelation takes in the narrative. As argued by Laura Mulvey and illustrated in the distinction between *Still Alice* and *A Late Quartet*, the masculine melodrama traditionally results in reconciliation and the female melodrama combines emotional excess (not entirely relevant to *Still Alice*) and unresolved contradictions.[20]

The transformative power of the diagnosis provides a narrative engine as it sets adrift multiple partnerships within the quartet. The medical problem becomes an emotional, a social, and a creative one for the three other members. Mitchell becomes the one who needs to soothe the tensions within the quartet, rather than being the one around whom the others gather. In this, and other examples where the character accepts the diagnosis, the character accesses a form of wisdom and

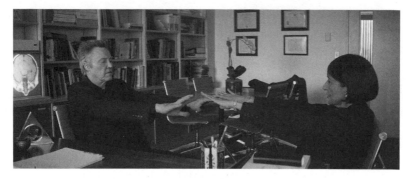

5.2 Peter Mitchell (Christopher Walken) with his doctor (Madhur Jaffrey), before the diagnosis of Parkinson's disease, in *A Late Quartet*.

serenity (in a mode reminiscent of melodrama) in which acceptance of fate provides closure and resolution of narrative tensions.

This film has two diagnostic revelation sequences. Similar to *Still Alice*, there is one scene in a medical setting (figure 5.2) and another when the performer announces his diagnosis to the other members of the quartet. The physician is portrayed as a gentle and caring older general practitioner. She delivers her assessment on the basis of a simple physical examination and the patient's account of his experiences. While she does request further tests, she assures the Walken character that she has little doubt. The announcement of the diagnosis is so clearly unequivocal in the narrative that the film does not even confirm the announcement with the results of the further tests she proposes he undertake.

The second diagnostic announcement occurs when Mitchell shares the news with his long-standing collaborators. The meeting takes place in his elegant home, around a table. The soundtrack (a piece we can assume is meant to be from one of the quartet's recordings), as well as the editing (a series of shots where the other three members of the quartet engage in a conversation we cannot hear), suggest that Peter Mitchell observes his friends and collaborators, feels isolated from them, and bears the emotional weight of the announcement he is about to make. As in *Still Alice*, the character is shot in isolation, reflecting and observing his surroundings and those close to him. The first shot of the sequence shows in medium close-up, looking off-screen to the left of the frame, then lowering his eyes as if he were taking stock of the moment and the emotional and psychological weight of the pending announcement.

The sequence also emphasizes his dominance by using a few over-the-shoulder shots that frame his body in the foreground and while his friends talk among themselves, or while he is making his announcement and immediately afterward, they look at him. His revelation is emotionless and concise, and while he is aware of the impact of the news, he insists on taking control. Without preamble, he states: "I spoke with Dr Nadir. This difficulty I've been having, Parkinson's, she says, early stages, maybe." Then, as his collaborators start negotiating the gravity of his illness he retorts: "I need to be real about this. Deal with it. Name it." Finally, as they cannot grasp that this will have an immediate impact on their creative collaboration, he unambiguously makes them confront the inevitable: "I've made up my mind, it's best for the quartet to plan ahead, to think about what comes next."

Contrary to Alice, and in line with gender distinctions in melodrama, he keeps tight control of the narrative and is not willing to become the object of others' responses and management. While Alice's family starts discussing her as if she were not there, Peter Mitchell does not let others start negotiating the implications of his illness or the decisions he has made. The premise of the narrative and the nature of this inciting incident is that it is not the illness that needs negotiation and management (it is a given that everyone accepts the diagnosis) but rather, the social consequences of the disease on others. After the announcement of the diagnosis, the group's latent frictions erupt into full-blown conflicts, including between the married couple and the revelation that the third member was in love with the wife within that couple (even as he started sleeping with their daughter). As in *Still Alice*, the diagnosis becomes a narrative engine that reveals characters and brings to the fore conflicts and tension that threaten, even more than the illness of the musician, the existence of the quartet. At the darkest point in the film, the mere possibility that the members of the quartet could recover the intimate understanding and trust that has distinguished their group is under radical threat.

The film achieves closure and emotional and narrative balance through the transcending gesture and benevolence of the retiring and ill member of the quartet in distinctly melodramatic terms: the illness punctuates Walken's character's serenity and grace and redeems (narratively) the others. As in *Still Alice*, the ill character metaphorically, and in this instance, literally, walks off stage in a gesture of acceptance of his illness and its consequences and as a gift and redemptive offer to the others. Here, even more than in *Still Alice*, the diagnosis transforms the characters and their social relations in ways that are threatening and yet ultimately affirmative. Both *Still Alice* and *A Late Quartet* offer variations on this theme.

Wit[21] starts, like a number of films in this genre (like the television series *Breaking Bad*, in particular), with a diagnosis, but the diagnosis is in *media res*, that is to say, the beginning of the story precedes the beginning of the film. There might have been symptoms, concern, a series of medical tests, and a diagnostic process, but none of this is shown to the viewer; it is implied by the diagnostic scene that is in fact, the very first shot of the film.

Wit centres almost exclusively on the paradoxical intimacy of an intelligent, articulate, and successful female professor (diagnosed with ovarian cancer) with the medical institution into which she is thrust and with which she is in permanent resistance. The film's original form as a play remains visible in the treatment of space as *huis-clos*, which intensifies the inter-relation of institutional and personal tensions.

The film opens with a close-up of an oncologist whose face awkwardly enters the frame: the film has no establishing shot to provide a context, background information, a sense of the characters or the stakes. The first line of dialogue in the film is solemnly delivered by the physician: "You have cancer. Miss Bearing, you have advanced metastatic ovarian cancer." A reverse shot shows Vivian Bearing, caught in what looks like emotional suspension; in two medium close-up shots and one line of dialogue, the entire premise and dramatic tension of the film is revealed. This is, as in *Still Alice*, something of a convention of diagnostic sequences: the announcement does not seem to register immediately. The institutional setup for the diagnostic pronouncement insists.

Already implicit in this scene are the power relations of this situation: a male expert delivers a life-threatening diagnosis to a female patient. As if the power relations were not already overdetermined, the medium close-up which reveals Bearing catches her looking upwards, more stable in the frame than the doctor but also more passive and more vulnerable. Her response after a moment of silence, "Go on," marks the intensity of the moment and the ceremony-like occasion as the receiver of medical news. The next short exchange encapsulates the terms by which the gender and power tensions between these two different characters will play out: "You are a professor, Miss Bearing," he says in a tone that is more condescending than inquiring.

"Like yourself, Dr Kelekian," Bearing answers sullenly.

"Ah yes," he retorts as if surprised by her claim and as if the allowance he already made for her social and intellectual status was sufficient and did not require an answer. The semblance of her comparable status he concedes suggests that he trusts she can process the information, take a detached and objective view of the situation, and recognize that the power of evidence makes the prognosis ineluctable. His talking to her as if she were a peer is not as much about erasing the power imbalance inherent in the situation (one person holds life-transforming information over the other) as it is about her having to abide by the informed and authoritative position he occupies. However, the film repeatedly plays on collusion and similarity between likeness and unlikeness between these two characters and a series opposites. In her analysis of the play, Slomith Rimmon-Kenan writes:

> The complex balance between similarities and differences informing the relations between the two main spaces in the play, the hospital and the university, as well as their equivocal connection with the world of language and its manifestations in two opposed yet parallel intertexts, acquires a self-reflexive dimension in the play's attitude to the world of the theatre and the role Vivian undertakes in it. As if to regain the position of power she had had at the university and lost in the hospital, Vivian assumes the role of a narratorial agent (an "impresario," she says), self-consciously presenting the play to the audience, commenting on it, controlling and manipulating the spectators' reactions.[22]

In the filmic adaptation of the play, this narratorial agency is translated into the breaking of the fourth wall and Vivian Bearing talking directly to the camera, taking viewers as both witnesses and recipients of her professorial pronouncements and capacity to retain control of the narrative.

The rest of this opening sequence, centred on the diagnostic announcement, oscillates between moments where they share observations about the qualities of their respective students, or lack thereof, and the visible excitement he reveals when trying to convince her to enrol in a "very aggressive" and experimental new treatment: "the strongest thing we have to offer you." His research pitch relies not so much on the fact that the treatment might offer her some hope for the future, but rather that "as research it will make a significant contribution to knowledge," a statement that is at best an appeal to the inquiring mind of the professor of English, and at worst, an acknowledgment that her illness is a way of advancing his scientific ambitions. As Rimmon-Kenan suggests, the convergence of interests and commitments of the medical practitioner's research with that of the professor of English literature ripples through the narrative in a series of contrasts and oppositions, including the function of language and narrative as escapes from the constraining reality of the hospital. Ultimately though, "language in *Wit* is thus perceived as both an alternative to the world of the hospital and as similar to the very space it tries to transcend, gradually shrinking and ultimately helpless against pain and death."[23]

At the conclusion of the film, and despite the itinerary she and her medical carers have taken to both humanize her and for her to be at peace with her mortality, a young doctor finds her unresponsive and he calls for the resuscitation team, the code team. When a nurse who knows Bearing well implores that he stop resuscitation (she is "no code" – an expression of her will not to be revived), his answer is "she's research!" a statement that is paradoxical. It simultaneously confirms the diagnostic power relations against which she's constantly resisting, and her own previously voiced attempt to retain agency through research, a defining feature of being an academic, and through her narratorial agency via storytelling.

The opening sequence sets the pattern that unfolds during the film: her illness hampers her search for independence and personal achievement through professional success, the sharpness of her intellect, and her ability to stand against adversity. It is not so much the diagnosis that she contests through the film but the threat the illness poses to her determination and ambitions, and those who are supposed to use their professional skills and judgment to treat her. *Wit* explores the predicament implied in acquiescing to medical care and the inherent power relations. It is also through her diagnosis that she becomes "body." As Klaver writes:

Indeed, through surgery and other forms of treatment, disease concepts can literally etch themselves as signifiers on the flesh. Nowhere in *Wit* is this point more poignantly evidenced than in the split dialogue that occurs during Grand Rounds: at the bedside, Jason intones: "At the time of first-look surgery, a significant part of the tumor was de-bulked ... Left, right ovaries. Fallopian tubes. Uterus. All out." And on Vivian's side: "*they read me like a book.*"[24]

Even more than *Wit*, *Angels in America*,[25] also directed by Mike Nichols, explores the politics of illness. Based on a play written by Tony Kushner and premiered in 1993, the television series is set in 1985 and explores the AIDS crisis, the cultural and social negotiations around homosexuality, and the epidemic spread of AIDS. Just as *Wit* did, *Angels in America* mixes fantasy and reality. It also constructs a complex tapestry of characters whose lives intersect: some are based on actual persons; others are fictional. One of the characters is based on Roy Kohn, the notorious Republican lawyer who participated in the McCarthy hearings and was on the prosecution team in the Rosenberg trial. He also was instrumental in the election of Ronald Reagan in 1980. In 1985 he was disbarred for unethical behaviour.

In an early scene of the television series, the Roy Kohn character, performed by Al Pacino, is visiting his physician. The physician is building up to telling Roy Kohn that he is infected with AIDS: he does not pronounce the diagnosis itself but details the symptoms of the disease and its likely course, preparing to tell Kohn that he has AIDS. He makes references to a range of autoimmune responses, including some that the character is already experiencing. A medium close-up of the physician captures his careful negotiation of the diagnostic announcement he will end up reserving. The Kohn character responds belligerently and threateningly: "Why are you telling me this?" Contrary to all the previous examples used here, there is no deployment of shot/reverse shot, medium shots, and no registration of the impact of the diagnosis on the face of the Roy Kohn character, even in the form of a passive stare. He is shown from the perspective of the physician, in the background as he is dressing after the examination. He doesn't flinch, and there is no close-up of his face to suggest that he is even processing the information. This visually and narratively introduces the terms by which the scene will play itself out: the diagnosis of AIDS does not and cannot remain. Eschewing the diagnosis, the medical authority, the sick role, or more importantly, the homosexual connection to the sick role, is visually embodied in these out-of-balance shots: the physician is shown in medium close-ups in a diplomatic if not tortured performance; Roy Kohn is inscrutable in the medium long shot that shows him in a backroom.

The remainder of the sequence is an exchange between the physician and Roy Kohn who challenges his doctor to explain the possibility of an AIDS diagnosis, which only affects homosexuals as far as he is concerned. Even admitting that he has sex with men, Kohn denies that he is a homosexual and denigrates homosexuals as weak. The Kohn character not only contests the AIDS diagnosis but argues that it is not possible, given his own power and strength. For Kohn, his very being, his identity, makes it impossible for him to be a homosexual, regardless of his actual sexual orientation.

Kohn dares his doctor to confirm he is a homosexual by diagnosing him with AIDS, threatening him with professional destruction. In this case, there is a reversal of the authority we have seen embedded in the previous examples, with the patient having the upper hand. He will succeed in getting his physician to refer to his diagnosis as "liver cancer," which he will do with exasperation, a subterfuge viewers know was prevalent in the early days of the AIDS epidemic. Kohn's interruption of the diagnostic moment is an act of control and power, even though he does not contest the symptoms and their probable cause (the dynamics of the sequence makes it clear that he knows exactly what he has).

Angels in America captures the politics of disease and naming in the context of 1980s Reagan America: diagnosis is a form of power Roy Kohn is not willing to concede. As such, and in opposition to all other main characters described here, he is not willing to contemplate the power of diagnosis over his self-agency. This makes the character both an illustration of self-loathing homophobia in the most intense and personal way, and a paradoxical revelation of the power and significance of diagnosis. Diagnosis, as well as its denial, fuels an egotistical act of self-empowerment and rage.

The diagnostic scene is powerful and common in contemporary film and television, and it performs many functions in narrative. In this chapter, we have focused on films in which the main characters and protagonists are those being diagnosed. However, we could have just as easily focused on the physicians. A slew of programs and films use the diagnostic moment to shape narratives around, and characterizations about, medical characters. *House, MD*, as we described above, is one of the best-known example, where the main character's diagnostic skills are cast as forensic in nature: the dysfunctional detective/diag-nostician, in Sherlock Holmes's style, redeeming himself through his careful sleuthing to arbitrate diagnosis.

But we could also look at *Médecin de campagne*, a French film in which the doctor is both diagnostician and at the same time, diagnosed. The first scene of the film is not redolent of *Breaking Bad*, it is quasi-identical. The 50-something country doctor, Jean-Pierre Werner, listens to his own doctor and colleague drone on about Werner's diagnosis, in much the same way as does Walter White, in *Breaking Bad*.

DOCTOR: Jean-Pierre. Jean-Pierre. Do you understand what I just said?
WERNER: Umh. Left temporal tumor. Inoperable
DOCTOR: I am sorry, but I want to know if you understand.
WERNER: In the best of cases, with chemo, I might pull through.
DOCTOR: Yes. You must get someone to replace you. You have to stop
  work if you want a chance of getting better.
WERNER: You have ink, or coffee, or I don't know what (pointing at the
  doctor's white coat). [translation, ours]

In this film, as in *Breaking Bad*, the patient clings to the banality of the present by focusing on the stain on the doctor's jacket. The characters in both productions resist transformation, at least initially. In *Médecin de campagne*, however, Jean-Pierre Werner starts from the authoritative position of doctor himself. As patient, however, he must acquiesce to the higher power (his own doctor) and submit to his admonition to work less. Progressively, Werner will give in to this power: first hiring and second trusting a replacement doctor with whom he will share the tasks he has been single-handedly undertaking for so many years. She will assist him in his noble task of home visits, palliative care, and general community support. He will be rewarded for his submission, as he ends up cured. The diagnosis has allowed him to become a more sociable character and emerge from the disease better than he was be-fore, rather than to decline towards death, as does White.

Or there is *Side Effects*.[26] In this 2013 film, we see again, negotiation of authority and power, with the power imbalance initially leaning to-wards the calculating female patient, rather than towards an omnipo-tent physician. In this psychological thriller, the patient painstakingly constructs a case to establish her diagnosis of depression and her sub-sequent need for an anti-depressant whose side effects she knows to include somnambulism (sleep walking). She murders her husband but

makes it appear that she has done so unconsciously, during an episode of sleep walking. She threatens to destroy the psychiatrist who
prescribed the medication. In the end, he will regain the upper hand
by using the psychiatric diagnosis she herself had crafted to exculpate
her responsibility in her husband's murder as a means of keeping her
hospitalized, against her wishes, and medicated to the point of stupor.

These films and television shows all relate to patient (and impatient)
characters for whom the diagnostic moment acts as an inciting incident.
Within these films are issues of power and authority, conflict and acceptance, and filmic conventions that focus on (or alternatively reject)
the afflicted character in ways that capture the character's response,
or processing, and formal isolation. These films require the viewers to
observe the character's thinking by creating a space in the texture of the
film that calls for their empathy and measure of their emotional investment in the character's predicament and the narrative unfolding.

Space and slowness are inscribed as metaphor for the character's
processing and reflection and also for viewers' empathetic investment.
The diagnosis has, by definition, a social and psychological meaning.
In the examples discussed here, medical authority is not contested in
terms of the diagnosis as a scientific fact. When the diagnosis is contested, as in *Wit* and *Angels in America*, the contest is not based on
the medico-scientific ways of knowing but on the power relationships
between the doctor and the patient, and who can keep the upper hand
longest.

The moment of diagnosis, in all these examples, is a moment of loss.
To punctuate its transformational power, the characters enduring these
transformations need to fall from high. In all of these scenes, the protagonists are mainly white, middle to upper-middle class, and with a
lot to lose. That many are artists, professionals, physicians, teachers,
or professors underlines that they do not lack the capacity to face the
diagnosis in terms of financial, social, emotional, reflexive, and commu-
nicational means. It is exactly because they are so endowed in resources
that the challenge of a life-threatening diagnosis is an expression of fate
and a relinquishing of power.

Rare are the films in which a diagnostic pronouncement occurs in a
character already deprived in the way all the other characters discussed
here are not. The most striking of these examples is Alejandro González
Iñárritu's *Bíutiful* in which the main character is diagnosed with terminal prostate cancer while his already precarious existence collapses
in a series of dramatic events. While trying to organize the life of his

children in anticipation of his death, he makes one poor decision after another. He is responsible for the death of many Chinese illegal workers. The African woman to whom he entrusted the care of his children and gave all his money, flees. While the film concludes with the prospective carer of his children changing her mind and returning to fulfil her promise, the film focuses less on the experience of illness and the injustice of fate than on the dislocation and the social precarity of the main character and his relationship with migrant workers in a society rife with social injustice and exploitation.[27] Diagnosis is but one more destabilizing phenomenon among a litany of others.

In the films described in this chapter, the revelation of the diagnosis is a narrative beginning, much as it might be in everyday life, where the name of the diagnosis comes to organize symptoms, and make sense of disarray.[28] The diagnosis, whether the characters accept as such or fight against as an act of individual affirmation and resistance, is the beginning of the story.

Some films use the diagnosis to conclude a narrative, to tie up all the loose ends. A notable example of this, and importantly not from traditional American cinema, is Agnès Varda's *Cléo From 5 to 7* which narrates, over the 90-minute film, two hours during which a woman awaits her 7 o'clock doctor's appointment where she thinks she is going to find out she is seriously ill.[29] Like other films we described, this one also begins in *media res*, in the middle of a Tarot reading session that Cléo is attending while awaiting her doctor's appointment. The fortune teller reveals the death card. The viewer has no idea why Cléo has gone to the doctor, and why it might have led her to see a fortune teller, but while she is awaiting the verdict from her doctor, she has received this ominous omen. We then follow her over the course of two hours, where the tension builds around this great uncertainty and her restlessness.

The film ends, after a *flânerie* through Paris, when the doctor tells her that she has cancer and that treatment must start urgently.[30] The scene itself is remarkable among all the examples of films with diagnostic announcement. Cléo arrives at the hospital at the time she has been told to come, just as her doctor is in his sports car, getting ready to leave. He has forgotten her appointment, just as she has waited all day for it. He abruptly informs her companion – who isn't a life partner, just someone she's picked up while she is impatiently waiting, and curiously, whose life is also in suspended animation, as he is a soldier on leave – in the parking lot, and her life will change forever.

In this counter-example, where the diagnosis serves as closure (it's the last scene of the film and the protagonist finds solace in the announcement), the viewer is, like Cléo, relieved to finally find out what's happening, even if the diagnosis is bad. This film, like the others we have analysed above, punctuates the power of the diagnostic moment to perform numerous narrative functions in film and in cinema, just as it does in the life of the patient receiving a serious diagnosis.

Other examples of using diagnosis as, or in place of, denouement include the Hitchcock classic *Psycho*[31] in which a psychiatrist delivers a courthouse diagnosis about Norman Bates's split personality, and another French film, *I've Loved You So Long*,[32] in which the diagnostic revelation at the end explains the otherwise inexplicable behaviour of the main protagonist throughout the film. In *Psycho*, the diagnosis hardly stands for an explanation in the narrative: the visual and narrative treatment of the sequence scene is ironic. Any simple pronouncements aimed at explaining Norman Bates's murderous actions is a symptom of our ability to understand the depths of evil. In *I've Loved You So Long*, the revelation of the diagnosis at the conclusion retrospectively explains the perceived criminal acts of a desperate mother and as noted her untold and unrecognized sacrifice until the films' denouement.

One of the intriguing spectatorial and individual responses to these diagnostic pronouncements-as-denouement is the extent to which the revelations add an extra layer of complexity to the character or to the thematic concerns of the film or somehow provide an instrumental and artificial way out of a narrative predicament. The result is the viewer's potential sense of being manipulated, of the emotional and affective investment in the narrative being vacuous.

The films we have discussed here provide examples of the different ways of thinking about diagnosis and its relation to filmic and televisual narratives. While these stories draw on the emotional investment of the viewer and their familiarity with the rules of visual storytelling, they are not documentaries and not to be measured for their accuracy. Believability and accuracy are not the same: it does not matter if Walter White's diagnosis, his treatment, or the evolution of his illness fits medical textbook and academic expectations or not. What matters for most viewers is the fact that the diagnosis and the illness contribute to the transformation and the revelation of the character and that they feel some investment in following this progression. In most narrative cinema and television, elements of the plot (the announcement of illness) must count and add to the emotional and affective texture of the film.

This texture is what gives "realness" to them, in which, when the film is successful, we may end up convinced that this is what it's like, that these diagnostic scenes are examples of medicine, doctors, and their interactions with patients.

Yet it is not necessarily so, because these scenes are creative representations and have their primary function in the unfolding of the narrative. Their representation is not so much to show what it is to be a doctor and what it is to receive a diagnosis. It is situated at a different level. To operate effectively in narrative, the diagnostic scene must appeal to socially recognizable structures, like diagnostic power, sacrifice, or denouement, both in film and television and outside of it. It must also respond to the conventions of cinematic and television storytelling: characters are revealed by action; the diagnostic moments constitute initiation of the transformative journeys of the characters. The diagnostic moments need to have some kind of emotional pay-off for the characters and the viewers; they must affect us.

Films and television create a convincing sense of reality, so convincing, indeed that medical educationalists use diagnosis films for their value in portraying disease, the patient-doctor relationship, and beliefs about illness.[33] And, at another extreme, there is a "cinematherapy" movement, which touts the use of films as treatment. Like its partner "bibliotherapy" (which uses fiction for the same purpose) the focus of this movement is on how these creative portrayals offer a means for reflecting on life, its struggles, and its joys. We certainly believe that all things in life should give one pause, but our interest in the diagnostic moment in film is anchored elsewhere beyond measuring the accuracy of the representation of the experience of illness and the moment of diagnosis or the use of stories as dependable mood-altering tools for therapeutic self-management.

As we look at the narrative role of diagnosis in film and television, we are more interested in the way they punctuate conventions. Each diagnostic moment highlights recognizable social values, well beyond the individual scene, about gender, knowledge, class, the role of the professions, institutions, and more. These are the elements of narrative and of diagnosis that films reveal. They reveal the investment we (storytellers and viewers) make in stories for finding significance in the events of our lives.

CHAPTER SIX

A Picture Paints a Thousand Words:
The Graphic Diagnosis

with Ian Williams

Like the films and television shows discussed in chapter 5, cartoons, comics, and graphic novels may use diagnosis as a tool for telling stories, leaving their readers in suspense, or making them laugh. In this chapter, I have reproduced a series of images from Ian Williams's graphic novel *The Bad Doctor* to show how diagnosis can create characters, insert doubt, and emphasize the sometimes uncomfortable power of being a doctor. The graphic diagnosis is fictitious and entertaining but at the same time very serious; it punctuates important social issues in diagnosis and in the practice of medicine. In the pages that accompany these images, we will discuss both the representation of these social issues and how graphic novels and visual storytelling can play an important role in health care delivery.

Cartoons are a helpful way of getting a joke. They often point a finger directly at the punch line, showing a reader when it's time to laugh (or cry). There's a picture, along with the words, and it's static, so viewers can take their time. The characters won't change expression until the viewer's eyes drift to the next frame.

Of course, I personally enjoy medical and particularly diagnosis cartoons; at least I understand the topic, if not the humour. The points they usually choose to parody are the same ones I pick apart in my theoretical readings. For them to be funny, they have to focus on issues that either trouble, or are familiar to, their readers. The cartoons underline, in a different way from my scholarly readings, the role of diagnosis in

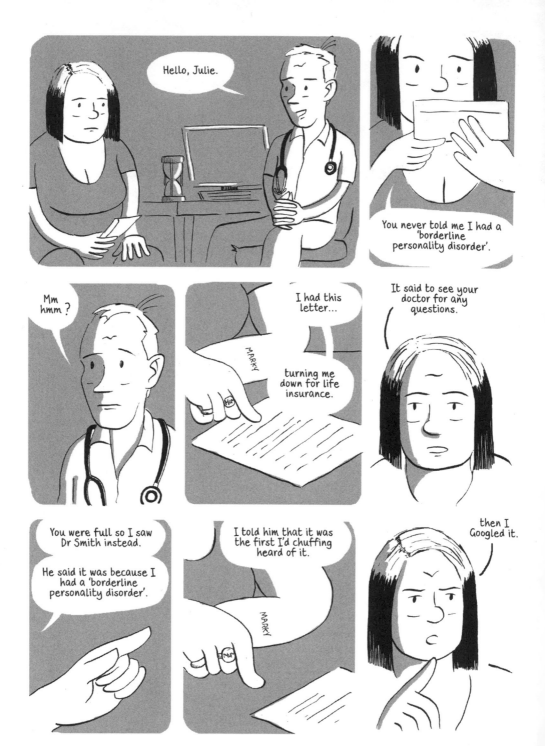

6.1–6.8 Julie's diagnosis. [Pages 38–45 reproduced with permission from *The Bad Doctor* by Ian Williams © Myriad Editions Ltd., London, 2014; Penn State University Press, PA, 2015.]

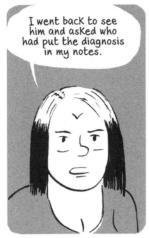

I went back to see him and asked who had put the diagnosis in my notes.

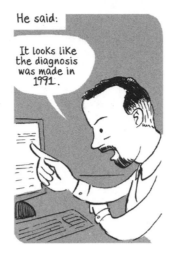

He said:

It looks like the diagnosis was made in 1991.

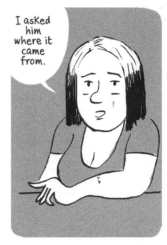

I asked him where it came from.

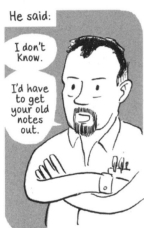

He said:

I don't know.

I'd have to get your old notes out.

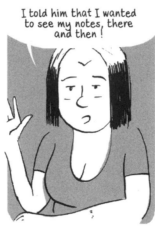

I told him that I wanted to see my notes, there and then!

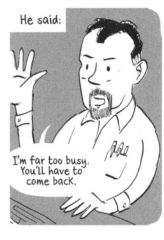

He said:

I'm far too busy. You'll have to come back.

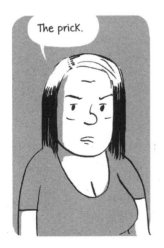

The prick.

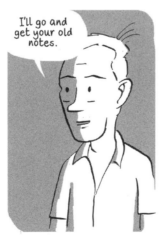

I'll go and get your old notes.

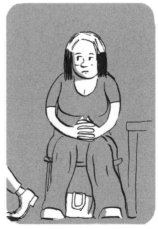

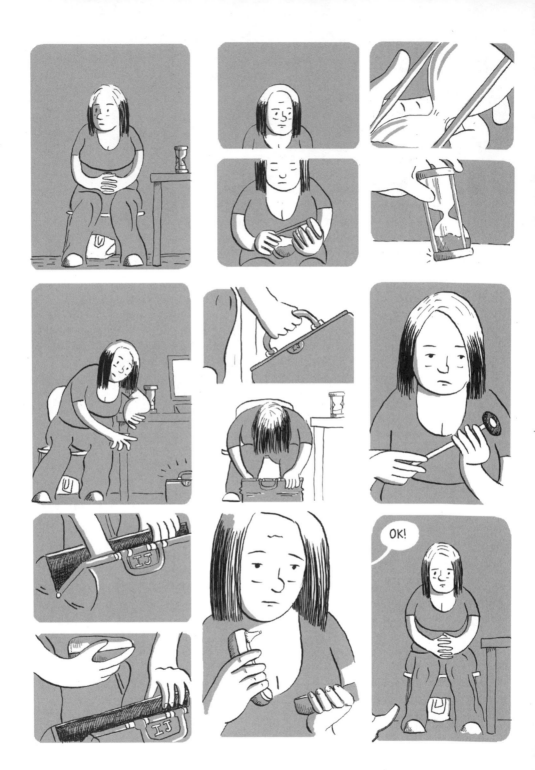

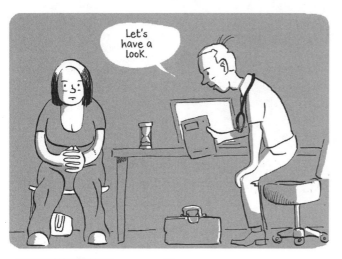

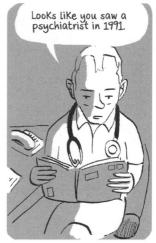

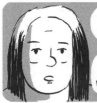

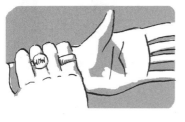

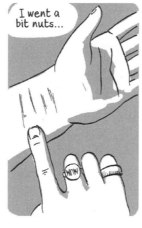

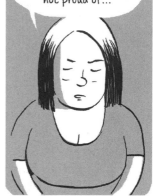

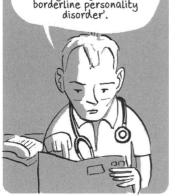

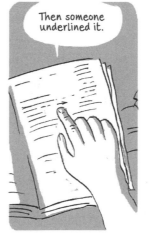

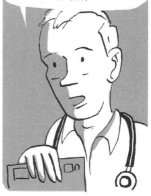

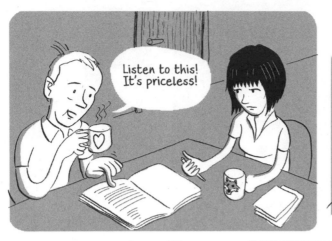

Listen to this! It's priceless!

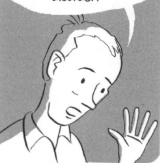

'She is a rather difficult and unpleasant woman who may, I suspect, have a borderline personality disorder.'

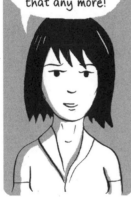

Consultants don't write letters like that any more!

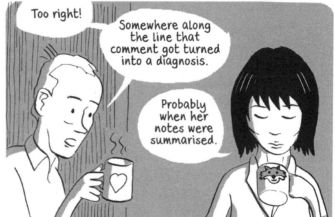

Too right!

Somewhere along the line that comment got turned into a diagnosis.

Probably when her notes were summarised.

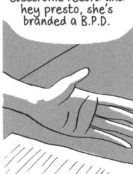

Then it got Read Coded and put on her electronic record and hey presto, she's branded a B.P.D.

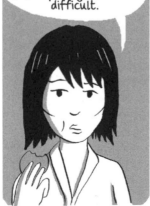

She is pretty weird and difficult.

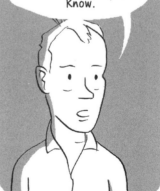

Well, yes, but no more so than a lot of people we know.

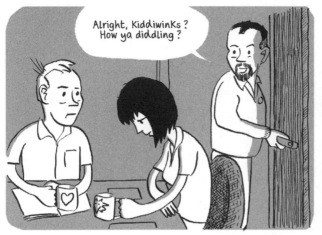

Alright, Kiddiwinks? How ya diddling?

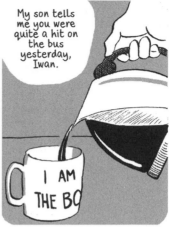

My son tells me you were quite a hit on the bus yesterday, Iwan.

I AM THE BO

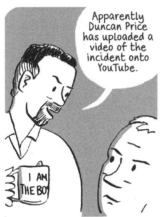

Apparently Duncan Price has uploaded a video of the incident onto YouTube.

I AM THE BO

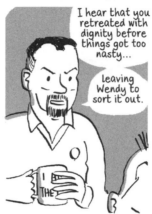

I hear that you retreated with dignity before things got too nasty...

Leaving Wendy to sort it out.

THE

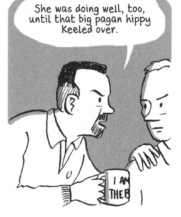

She was doing well, too, until that big pagan hippy keeled over.

I AM THE B

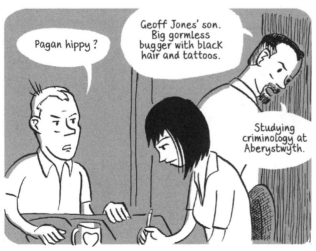

Pagan hippy?

Geoff Jones' son. Big gormless bugger with black hair and tattoos.

Studying criminology at Aberystwyth.

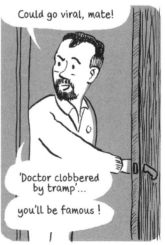

Could go viral, mate!

'Doctor clobbered by tramp'...

you'll be famous!

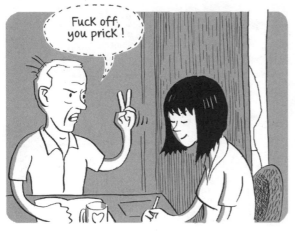
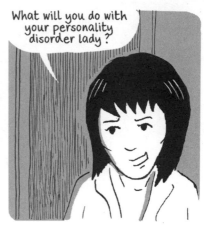
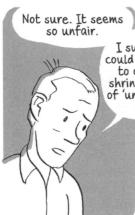
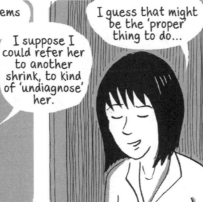
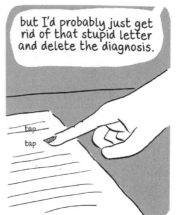
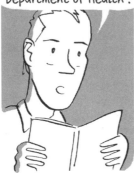
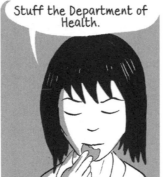
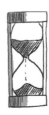

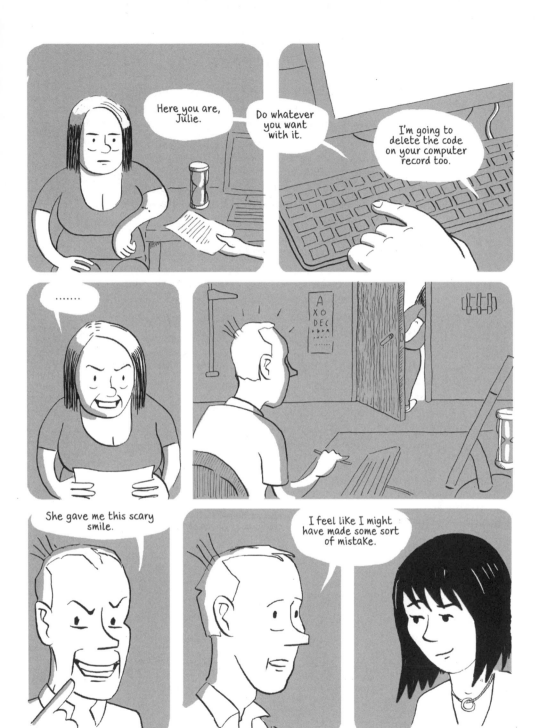

society. This is not to say that cartoons depict diagnosis the way it really is; they depict it in a way with which readers can connect. And as this book has highlighted throughout its pages, diagnosis is a logical topic for graphic artists, so common a Western trope it is for understanding human existence. Not only the *New Yorker*, but the *Guardian*, the *New York Times*, and the *Sydney Morning Herald* (to name only a very few) all frequently feature cartoons which either tell stories about diagnosis or use diagnosis to make particular points about the drama of human existence.

The use of graphic art to tell stories about diagnosis goes beyond the broadsheets and glossy coffee table magazines. It is used in patient teaching documents, notably for children. *Iggy and the Inhalers* features superhero inhalers such as Broncho, the rodeo bronchodilator, and Coltron, the transformer-robot anti-inflammatory inhaler who unite to combat the asthma triggers (Moldar, Pollenoid, Smoky Joe, and Hairy) all the while teaching children about the pathophysiology and treatment of asthma.

I met the author of this chapter via twitter. He was interested in my work on diagnosis, and I was interested in his on graphic medicine. Both a doctor and an artist, he contributes regularly to the *Guardian* with his medical cartoons, and developed the term *graphic medicine* in 2010, a movement that now has a substantial following (more on this shortly). Ian and I both inhabit the twittersphere, so it was just a matter of time before our paths would cross. I asked Ian about his favourite diagnosis scene from his own graphic story *The Bad Doctor*, and he sent me the pages that you have just read.

In this sequence, a patient named Julie confronts Dr Iwan James, her regular GP, about a diagnosis she didn't know she had:

> "You never told me I had a 'borderline personality disorder.' I had this letter ... turning me down for life insurance. It said to see your doctor for any questions."

I followed up, asking Ian why he had decided to write about the diagnosis of borderline personality disorder. He explained that he once had a patient himself who had received that diagnosis on the basis of a throwaway comment in a psychiatrist's letter. The comment had become written in stone, and the patient had come back to him to express her displeasure. He continued: "I wanted to make Julie's character slightly 'tricky' and wanted the narrative to be slightly ambiguous, so we don't quite know whether Iwan is being fooled or not." Ian has written elsewhere that "comics have a particular role to play in the discussion of difficult, complex or ambiguous subject matter."[1]

I was not surprised that Ian had chosen this particular diagnosis and this type of story for his graphic novel. For a number of reasons, borderline personality disorder creates a very good story for a graphic depiction of diagnosis. Julie's narrative illustrates how borderline personality disorder stigmatizes her and casts her in an undesirable light: she has become officially and pathologically obnoxious. It's a barrier to her future fulfilment, not because her life term is shortened or her lifestyle must be altered; her social prospects have been interfered with because of the diagnosis. Her routine expectations of being able to have life insurance or, possibly, apply for a job of some sort, have been messed with because someone put this diagnosis in her chart, as it appears, with cavalier insouciance.

And Julie never even knew she had been diagnosed. That is, until the secret was revealed by her rejected life insurance application. In contrast to many of the diagnostic scenes we have discussed previously, for Julie, the diagnostic moment took place in her absence. Had she been there, she might have been able to debate, contest, or clarify, that "negotiation" about which Balint wrote.[2] Julie didn't get to negotiate.

This graphic sequence underlines the important tensions in the diagnostic labelling process. Julie is powerless, both because of her previous ignorance of the diagnosis (she never even heard her diagnosis so couldn't reconcile herself to the label) and because the power to diagnose is located with the doctor, not the patient. One might protest that the increasing practice of self-diagnosis and the development of self-diagnosis tools and apps are making inroads to correcting this imbalance, but, well, not really. People can come to their doctors with a diagnosis in mind; they can be less submissive, armed as they are today with their Internet research and diagnostic proposals; and they can diagnose themselves and treat for a range of afflictions where medical resources aren't required (e.g., a self-diagnosed gluten-intolerant can remove gluten from her diet without medical assistance). However, the health care system can, and does, prevent patients from having diagnostic authority.

The Read Code referred to in the comic excerpt was the mechanism by which Julie's diagnosis was officially recognized in a medical record, and it is a code that only Julie's doctor can enter. Whether the coding system is SNOMED, DSM, ICD, or any one of the hundreds of coding tools available for counting, linking, and correlating diseases, the patient doesn't get to enter the code or alter it once it's cemented into place.[3] In Julie's case, it's not even clear that her own doctor can erase this code. It's as if she's branded for life. Dr James may be able to take the code out of her records, but when she goes to reapply for health insurance, she is likely to have to answer the question, Have you ever been turned down for insurance in the past? Her putative border-line personality disorder will rear its head again.

So, the diagnostic moment is a point of power, and at the same time, it is a point of tension, linked as it is with resource allocation (life insurance). The tension results from the fact that the doctor is the gatekeeper and therefore a potential point of resistance. For Julie, having a diagnosis is the problem; for other patients, not having one might be. Many diagnoses create tension between patients and their clinicians, either, as for Julie's, because the diagnoses are undesirable for the patient, or because the doctor is reluctant to believe in the diagnosis itself or that the patient has the given diagnosis. Joseph Dumit has written eloquently about "diagnoses you have to fight to get,"[4] and has typified these points of tension as being common in non-specific conditions for which there isn't a clear clinical marker.

It's true that diseases without their own lab tests often raise the loudest debates. This is because, as John Gardner explains, lab tests become the *arbiters* of diagnosis, taking a prominent place in the diagnostic process, despite their own fallibility and limitations.[5] Lab tests require context, and are often meaningless without. For example, *Neisseria meningitidis*, which is the bacteria that causes meningococcal disease, can live happily in the nasal passages of individuals who are not and will never become sick. It can also cause fatal bacterial meningitis and sepsis. The presence of the bacteria alone isn't enough to diagnose meningococcal meningitis.

In many conditions, normal markers or microbes are sometimes just normal and other times, diagnostic. It's not always problematic, but sometimes it is! The bacteria *G. vaginalis* can be in the genital tract of a woman who is perfectly fine or be diagnostic of bacterial vaginosis. For diabetes, hypertension, and overweight, cut-off points will determine whether a blood glucose level, blood pressure reading, weight, or other lab value indicates disease or normal function. Why is a systolic blood pressure of 139 normotensive and of 140 hypertensive? In any case, there are no blood tests for mental illness, and this in and of itself puts psychiatric diagnoses into the very-likely-to-be-contestable category.

This brings us back to what we discussed in chapter 1: diseases are not as certain as they appear at first blush. Their boundaries are porous, negotiable, and debatable even when there is a laboratory test. But despite all their uncertainty, there is, as Julie's case illustrates, certainty of effect in both the medical and the individual narrative. Is Julie's story one of the wronged wife who discovers her husband in bed with her friend and goes "a bit nuts," or is it one of an unstable woman with psychiatric risk factors? It depends on whose narrative we are reading. This is an example of what Frank refers to as "a *narrative surrender*" in which the good patient relinquishes her story to the doctor.[6] The doctor retells this story through diagnosis, and the new narrative becomes "the one against which others are ultimately judged true or false, useful or not."[7] In Julie's story, there is a progressive and increasing surrender in which her story is diluted and mediated at each step until it becomes unrecognizable to her.

The Read Code is ultimately the device by which her story is transformed. Julie's diagnosis was initially proposed as a question ("might have borderline personality disorder"), it was underlined by an unidentified "someone," but once the diagnostic code is entered into her records, she has a new narrative, one of psychiatric risk.

Dr James, in a way, acknowledges, simultaneously, his power and his personal uncertainty, as he comments on her "scary" smile after he tells her he has removed the code that has given her the diagnosis. He may have made a mistake, he tells his colleague. Maybe she does have borderline personality disorder after all, but he has made it disappear. Dr James is a self-doubting superhero. He knows that he can, with a strike of the pen, rewrite her narrative. What he doesn't know, and may never find out, is whether or not he has told it the right way.

Ian himself, as I said above, has maintained that graphic medicine, or the use of comics and graphic novels, has great potential to help carers, health professionals, and patients themselves understand the experience of health, illness, and of course diagnosis. Since his call in 2010 for graphic medicine, there has been an influx of interest, with increasing exploration of what comics have to offer medicine.

Cartoons provide a valuable visual tool that many have been keen to harness for the purpose of patient education, particularly the education of children. Comic strips have been developed to help children understand research and informed consent,[8] to explain treatments,[9] to promote screening initiatives,[10] and to provide views of illness to medical students that differ from the traditional medical curriculum.[11]

That the graphic medium can serve educational purposes is worth noting. For the same reasons that it can be easier to get a joke when it is told via frames, a cartoon offers a different medium for conveying information and, as such, has the potential to help an individual understand and process complex information. In this context, comics are didactical, developed with a particular aim in mind.

However, beyond the on-purpose construction of educational material via graphic novels, we can consider their construction as stories per se: not stories of diagnosis or stories trying to document a lived reality. They are stories that are drawn to entertain, using familiar constructs and characters that readers can follow; they generate a creative imaginary. They are not concerned with what doctors should or shouldn't do in a clinical setting or what it is "like" to have a particular diagnosis. Rather, they implement all the tools of storytelling, such as pathos, emotions, and humour towards a narrative end. The "what if" of narrative is not the same as the "what if" of medical diagnosis. Readers respond to the circumstances via their knowledge of storytelling and how they might refract reality. By *refract* I mean that the starting point, real as it might be, is broken and reassembled to create a narrative component which stimulates interest.

I turn to the comic hero par excellence, Superman, to complete this discussion. In a grave scene depicted in All-star, Superman is told that he is suffering from "apoptosis." There is no pretense, in the scene, to educate or to document the experience of illness, but rather to produce a narrative turn where Superman's mortality and the continuation of his projects are emphasized. This diagnosis, which is not completely fictitious (apoptosis refers to a pathophysiological process that exists in humans, albeit at a cellular level) provides a backdrop for the angst and energy that Superman will need to preserve humanity from evil.

Even while superman's apoptosis is not intended as an opportunity for medical education, it incorporates diagnosis in the story in a way that is recognizable to readers and gives them pause. It contributes further to a superman metaphor of strength against all odds. The diagnosis of apoptosis contributes to Superman's mystique and to ways of engaging with the world. What makes this example poignant is that Superman's diagnosis is shaped differently from in the prevalent templates; his diagnosis highlights his character and his role, rather than transforms them. We will return to this in chapter 8. *All-Star Superman* is not an illness narrative; it is purely fiction. But it is not unbridled; it is, as we described, a *refraction*, a reaction to the creative potential of diagnosis.

CHAPTER SEVEN

The Intellectual Documentary: Methods for Understanding the Diagnostic Moment

It is through stories of diagnosis that we can both understand our reactions and reclaim them; there is powerful potential in popular narratives. Diagnosis, as much as disease, bullies its way into our life or the lives of people around us and claims a chunk of it. But, at the same time, it becomes a rudder which gives us direction in uncharted waters, answering questions about what's happening, what can be done, and what the future looks like. The potential of diagnosis is, in any case, transformative: disruptive and destructive or alternatively explanatory and prophetic. Shifting the balance away from the destructive transformative power of the diagnosis requires re-narration and introspection, actions that the personal illness narrative genre has generated.

Suzanne Fleischman's illness narrative provides the title to this chapter. She wrote an essay at the end of the last century which has been important to my understanding of the social functions of diagnosis. She called this essay a "documentary," and in it she made a short statement that changed the direction my scholarly diagnosis work had taken, moving it towards the development of this book. Suzanne was a linguist at the University of California Berkeley in the 1990s. Diagnosed with a rare, and ultimately fatal haematological disorder, Fleischman reflected upon her condition. More specifically, she tried to develop from her own experience a more generalizable exercise in medical semantics, using her training as a linguist to explore how language shapes the experience of illness and disease.[1]

Writing with her own diagnosis as a starting point, Fleischman explained, "If a person is told 'you have cancer' (or any life-threatening disease) *these words* irrevocably alter that person's consciousness, view of the future, relationship with family and friends, and so on. Moreover, the utterance marks a boundary. It serves to divide a life into 'before' and 'after,' and this division is henceforth superimposed onto every rewrite of the individual's life story."[2] It was these words that pushed me towards writing about and trying to understand the diagnostic moment and its narratives.

At the time she wrote her paper, the "illness narrative," or the widely published patient accounts of illness, was on the rise even though it was not a new tradition. As Art Frank, author of numerous scholarly works on the illness narrative, has pointed out, it was in 1623 that John Donne wrote "Devotions upon Emergent Occasions" in which he described how his illness brought him a new perspective to his religious faith.[3] However, since the last few decades of the twentieth century, there has been an impressive upswing in publication of accounts of illness by the people experiencing the illness, rather than by their doctors or unaffected observers. It is a kind of contemporary genre, wrote Frank, that "represents one way of living *for* the other ... Storytelling is *for* an other just as much as it is for oneself."[4] The telling of stories about illness is important to the person who is ill, as these stories "sustain a relational self that is threatened by some crisis."[5]

The rise in the illness narrative is a combination of acceptance and of revelation, a storying in which the author "flaunts bodily conditions they might once have hidden, or camouflaged in fiction. Illness and disability memoirs have achieved great popularity, critical esteem, and currency in contemporary media. Along with gay, queer, and transgendered people, ill and disabled people are coming out in life writing."[6] Thinking of illness narratives as a "coming out" is another way to recover the self, rather than relinquish it to its diagnosis. It enables the author to establish the terms of the tale, shaping its representation and directing its plot. Via the illness narrative, the story can become one about living rather than about death, about self rather than about disease.

Particularly in an era of self-publishing, there are innumerable examples of eloquent writers who present the personal experience of illness to a broad public. Some of the most recent ones at the time this book goes to press include Jenni Diski, who wrote the serialized account of her lung cancer in the *London Review of Books*. Neurosurgeon Paul

Kalaninthi wrote *When Breath Becomes Air*, describing his diagnosis and decline from terminal cancer.[7] Amy Boeksy's edited *The Story Within* captures a range of personal perspectives on genetic diagnosis.[8]

However, Fleischman's goals were somewhat different. While she did locate her essay in her personal experience of illness, she used it to meld the analytic tools of her discipline with the human perspective of a patient. Fleischman may have felt the need for self-preservation that Frank identifies above but was also intent upon taking her personal experience of illness and imposing a critical intellectual analysis of the experience in linguistic terms. Her essay would be a case study of the semantics of diagnosis and illness, and a means for making sense of her individual experience and of the American health system.

Fleischman is not alone in making use of her personal experience for scholarly ends, and it shouldn't be surprising. The context that leads to the rise of the personal illness narrative is the same for scholars, and it would be hard to think that an individual who has devoted her life to a particular critical way of seeing the world wouldn't do the same in relation to the personal epiphany of diagnosis. While Fleishmann has considered her diagnostic experience as a linguist, Mildred Blaxter has considered hers as a sociologist,[9] Havi Carel as a philosopher,[10] and Martha Stoddard Holmes as a cultural and literary scholar.[11]

Their reflections provide not only intellectual documentaries but also frameworks for considering the diagnostic narrative and its construction. They provide us with tools for understanding – and also for re-creating – storytelling frames around the diagnostic moment. In this chapter, I focus on the writings of these authors about their diagnoses to uncover the potential their ways of thinking have to offer us as we continue to ponder the power of the diagnosis and of the diagnostician. These authors provide us with alternatives to the conventional stories that weigh heavily on our shoulders, whether we be the person diagnosed or the diagnostician. What these women do through their narratives is to cement their enduring identities as scholars, thinkers, and living humans. Their narratives are a form of resistance.

Mildred Blaxter can be remembered as one of the earliest sociologists of diagnosis. In 1978, well before she would write her personal diagnosis narrative, this British sociologist wrote a seminal paper on the social aspects of diagnosis.[12] Using alcoholism as an example, she underlined the inadequate attention sociology paid to this important action/thing in medicine. Let me explain my lazy, forward-slash compound word. Blaxter highlighted that diagnosis existed both as a process (action) and as a category (thing). Both were, however, social objects, and she described how concepts of disease, of medicine and of classification intersected to create practical, rather than nosological, problems for concepts of disease.

Blaxter's intellectual documentary, however, was published in 2009. She wrote a paper for *Sociology of Health and Illness*, a journal she had helped to develop many years prior, the single-case study of P and her diagnostic journey to explore and finally identify adenocarcinoma of the lung. She *is* P, as she reveals in the introduction to her paper. Blaxter died of this disease in 2010 at the age of 85.

Blaxter's rationale for her single-case study is grounded in a sociology of the body as much as it is a sociology of diagnosis. "The body is endlessly 'doubled and redoubled' through a chain of simulacra," she writes, explaining how Western medicine ceases to "see" the body it seeks to cure; rather, it *represents* the body via the diagnostic imaging technologies and media which are not only more and more readily available, but which are multiplying. These technologies take snapshots of the body that are translated first into numbers or data, and second into diagnoses, or stories about what's going on. It's a continual chain of symptoms translated into meaning by the intermediary of an image (X-ray, CT, PET, and so on). The symptoms and even the images are represented and represented until the pieces fall into place and sense-making is achieved.

Many sociologists argued that the body "disappeared" in favour of virtual imaged realities of the patient, which transferred control to the hands of those who ordered, manipulated, and interpreted the diagnostic images.[13] Others suggested that these technologies did not necessarily rip control away from the visually imaged person, that instead, the patient was an active subject, rather than a passive object.[14]

Blaxter's case study set out to explore her place in this visually mediated diagnostic process, keeping careful notes, diagnostic test reports, scans, and doctors' letters during the 141-day diagnostic process from first routine X-ray to diagnostic confirmation. From a detailed list of "events" (e.g., "abnormality identified," "lung biopsy," "consultation with GP1 about symptoms in neck"), Blaxter develops her own argument about the place of the patient in the diagnostic process. It is one in which P/Blaxter participates in the co-production of diagnosis.

As a matter of fact, Blaxter's role was narrative, as she assembled the bits and pieces of diagnosis produced by diagnostic technology and various specialities. Her experience of the process of diagnosis was fragmenting:

> The body is divided up into different organs and systems, each of which has to be looked at separately and serially. However, within medicine, many of these will have different specialists, departments, outpatient clinics, places within a hospital, or even different hospitals.[15]

With each movement between diagnostic locations, Blaxter would provide a history to the new clinician who would be bringing in a different view of a particular part of her body. In her retelling, she would draw the fragmenting images and specialities back together – and perhaps, "differently" together – for the new clinician. Each image would have frozen a particular instant, a particular position of her body that needed to be woven back into a moving, active whole. Yet, at the same time, the fragmented images of the inside of her body shaped for Blaxter the experience of being ill and offered her a way of owning the experience, a sensation depicted in the historical poster (figure 7.1).

Blaxter's intellectual documentary offers some critical sense-making tools about the social aspects of the diagnostic process. These *social* aspects are quite different from the *psychosocial* factors that generally preoccupy the clinician. The latter are often most concerned with micro-level factors that influence the individual patient: patient entourage, support structures, work, and leisure settings. Blaxter's work, on the other hand, encourages the critical scholar to explore organizational factors, beyond the individual doctor and patient. In line with Blaxter's impressive body of sociological work, she positions her research concerns outside of her individual case of how P and P's doctors interact and focuses instead on "the nature of 'evidence' in a world where neither the individual doctor nor the patient, but rather the measurement and the image, were increasingly becoming the vehicle of decisions."[16]

While decision making may take place at the level of the individual clinician-patient dyad, frameworks and contexts for this decision making are positioned in institutions well beyond these individual actions. Protocols and formal guidelines, themselves buttressed by evidence-based practice; multidisciplinary team systems, and inter-specialty social conventions are points at which social forces shape the diagnostic

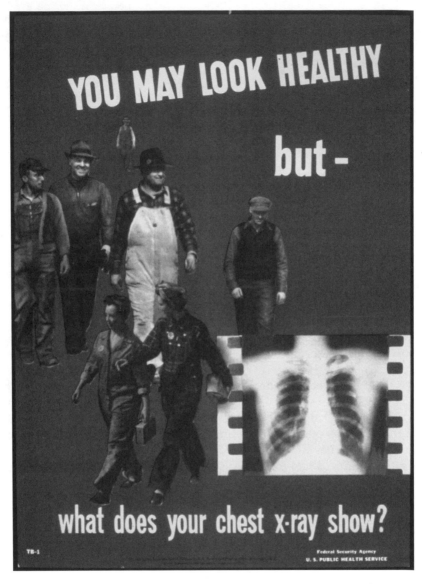

7.1 X-rays and diagnostic imaging creates a representation of a fragmented inner self. [Office for Emergency Management. Office of War Information. Domestic Operations Branch. Bureau of Special Services. (03/09/1943 - 09/15/1945). Credit: [Public domain], via Wikimedia Commons]

process. Their hierarchies, politics, power, influences, and histories are hidden from view but pivotal to the social understanding of diagnosis as experienced in Blaxter's case study. As she concludes "in modern medicine it is much more important for sociology to study what Cussins called the 'ontological choreography' of these ever more complex systems, including the way in which images and records appear to create and control both medical practice and the patient's medical experience. This is what actually counts."[17]

How do words work in the experience of diagnosis? What are the linguistic ramifications of how we talk about disease? Suzanne Fleischman uses her personal experience of the haematological disorder *myelodysplasia syndrome* as a starting point for exploring the "linguistic construction" of disease. Fleischman was a professor of linguistics in the department of French at the University of California (Berkeley).

In 1993, she received her diagnosis, as she explains it, as "a quirk of fate."[18] As I described in the opening paragraphs to this chapter, Fleischman experienced her own diagnosis as transformative. She was seemingly excellent health, but "out of the blue, my life plan was radically altered, my future thrown into question"[19] she wrote. As a linguist seeking to make sense of her own experience, she wrote this paper to reveal "the meanings and metamessages tucked away in the recesses of … language."[20]

Fleischmann, unlike the other authors included in this chapter, points out, as I did in chapter 1, the fluid nature of diagnostic categories. To say that one has this diagnosis or that diagnosis is not necessarily to be clear about the exact nature of the ailment. Myelodysplastic syndrome is an umbrella diagnosis that captures numerous types of disorders. While the differences may be significant, patients have only one way of speaking about their illness. In this composite category, the diagnostic term obfuscates rather than clarifies what ailment afflicts the individual. The name matters, writes Fleischman. It confers existence by "creat[ing] a 'thing' to which one can subsequently make reference, out of the seamless data of the physical and experiential world."[21].

But in the case of myelodysplastic syndrome, the name is barely recognizable outside of the specialized world of haematology, explains Fleischmann and that is because of the rarity of the diagnosis. "You have *my-low*-what?" squeal her interlocutors when her disease comes up in conversation.[22] In the absence of lay consciousness of a particular diagnosis or its features, the diagnosis fails to provide a sense of identity or of community, both expected outcomes of the diagnosis.

Disease is, at the same time, a collective and an individual experience. Fleischman punctuates this with a discussion of the illness-disease dichotomy. Illness is how the people feel in themselves – physically, emotionally, functionally, and dysfunctionally – while diseases are "conceptual entities, categories of clinical taxonomy."[23] These distinctions are reproduced in syntax, where the relationship of the individual to her pathology is embedded in the way she speaks about her illness and her disease ("I am diabetic" versus "I have diabetes" or "I suffer from diabetes").

Parts of speech provide shape to the way we can talk about diagnosis. The noun makes of disease a more solid object, gives it a more ontological existence and more concrete boundaries than – as I exposed in chapter 1 – are actually the case. But nouns do more than this, explains Fleischman:

> Nouns congeal what is essentially a process into a static state that becomes superimposed on the individual rather than the individual being construed as an integral part of the development of the disease.[24]

Verbs, on the other hand, are more frequently associated with the process of acquiring of disease and tend to be both euphemistic and passive. *Falling ill, getting* (or *taking*) *sick, coming down* with something, leave the individual out of the equation, while *catching* a cold implies a bit of participation, as if the person should have prevented the infection. Fleischman refers to these as "inceptive" verbs and ponders how they symbolically demarcate the transformative power. When does one *get, come down with*, or *catch* progressive diseases such as her myelodysplastic syndrome, when the onset of the pathology is often well in advance of any symptoms? The utterance is the moment one becomes aware, when the impact is made, but not the moment at which the disease is acquired. As a linguist, Fleischman also underlines the many metaphors of battle which are reserved for bad diseases which "strike" us.

The question of metaphor is one which had been previously raised, and dealt with by Susan Sontag in her seminal *Illness as Metaphor*.[25] It was in 1978, facing a cancer diagnosis of her own, that Sontag decried the battle metaphors that dominated her (and other) clinical discussions of cancer in particular but illness in general. A literary theorist, she demonstrated the degree to which ill-chosen metaphors create fantasies about diseases and add greatly to patient suffering. Her book was also about reclaiming. She explained that "the healthiest way of being ill – is the one most purified of, most resistant to, metaphoric thinking … It is toward an elucidation of those metaphors, and a liberation from them, that I dedicate this inquiry."[26]

Euphemism, as well, contributes to the linguistic construction of diagnosis. Given the transformative power of the diagnostic utterance that Fleischman has so aptly described, and rendered more powerful still because of her dual position as diagnosed and as linguistic, euphemisms provide some mild dilution. In the same way that the diagnostic categories break the continuum of nature into manageable chunks (see, notably Zerubavel[27] on this), euphemisms make them *emotionally* manageable.

She also writes about the occupational registers that frame diagnosis. These registers are the way specialists talk among themselves but are not very helpful for people outside of the speciality. With respect to diagnostic language, there are interesting appropriations (and misappropriations!) of the technical language. Davison and his colleagues reported how laypeople adopted an epidemiological affect and language to describe disease risk, even when their explanations were far removed from those of the medical experts.[28]

What do patients understand of this foreign language, this occupational register? Do they start speaking like a tourist to Europe with school-girl French and no sense of the subtle cultural differences between speakers of English and French, or do they give up trying to understand, living instead in isolation in the small remnant of a world they do understand? This is particularly challenging when specialized terms in the medical world have other meanings in the vernacular. Fleischman explains that while "indolent" sounds like laziness to the layperson, in reference to a serious diagnosis, it's actually good news: the condition is moving slowly.

Fleischman underscores that whatever social meanings we give to a particular body part – heart, brain, marrow – will transfer over to diseases of those parts. She concludes: "When one suffers from a serious illness, the affected organ or body part is never *just* a body part. It carries multiple layers of culturally-determined associative meaning."[29]

Havi Carel is a professor of philosophy at the University of Bristol in the United Kingdom. She was diagnosed with a disease perhaps even more rare than Fleischman's called *lymphangioleiomyomatosis*. This disease with a 25-letter name was not one that lay dormant, discovered by a random blood test, it was one which was announced first by a significant change in Carel's functional abilities which incited her to seek medical attention. Her fitness faltered, she struggled to ride her bike, to climb stairs, to do those things she normally did with ease. In "With Bated Breath"[30] and *Illness*,[31] Carel describes how her diagnosis was pivotal to her experience of illness, but as much as the diagnosis was a disruptive and traumatic experience, it was also a moment at which new possibilities were opened to her.

As she describes her experience of illness, her discovery of disease, her perception of newly discovered limitations in her actions and in her future potential, she offers a philosopher's view of diagnosis which she goes so far as to describe (in Epicurean terms) as "therapeutic" – like a medicine. For Carel, diagnosis transforms the illness experience. No longer is it "a private musing on the nature of bodily change, but an item in a medical vocabulary and ontology, to which shared meanings and knowledge are attached."[32] And with this comes some of what we discussed in the introduction. There is a "sense of having an objective and known condition releases at least some of the sense of shame, guilt, and inadequacy that may characterize earlier stages of symptom experience."[33]

The transformative power of the diagnostic label is typically cast in terms of "closed possibilities" as so many of the narratives we have visited together either enunciate clearly or imply. It's the gavel, the scalpel, the enduring boundary between before and after. For Carel, it was that the "list of things given up and crossed off may become ever longer as time goes by, cementing the sense of closure. This was for a long time, the sole paradigm in descriptions of illness: loss, the breaking of identity, disruption of narrative, and disruption of lived experience."[34]

It is the link between diagnosis and prognosis that creates this closure; it is the notion that our days are limited. However, Carel points out that this was always already the case. It is the notion of finitude that shapes our life.[35] She draws on a range of models to illuminate this idea and to explore how diagnosis opens up possibilities in a life which was only ever going to be finite anyway.

Michel de Montaigne, the French renaissance philosopher and statesman wrote that the goal of philosophy was to learn how to face death with equanimity. Our contemporary way of living tends to encourage us to avert our thoughts from the problem of death. But the disease and its associated diagnosis puts the notion of death firmly in our view. It provides, according to Carel, an opportunity to live reflectively and achieve this philosophical goal.

Drawing upon both Heidegger, a twentieth-century phenomenologist, and the ancient Greek philosopher Epicurus, she presents us with models for accepting death, and for using diagnosis as a means by which we are achieve equanimity. The diagnosis opens us to vulnerability and to dependence, both of which provide us with possibilities for more fully experiencing our life. "Accepting that the human project is towards death, that death structures our life, we are freed up in in our ability to *be*."[36]

The Heideggerian approach that Carel presents is concerned with how death structures our life and shapes our existence. Every living moment "should be understood as unique, irreversible and as bringing us closer to death ... there are no second chances. I can never repeat today."[37] It is only in relation to its finitude that life makes any sense at all. Yet that finitude is often offered only to those who are forced to look at it, as, for example, in the revelation of a dire diagnosis. In this way, the diagnosis is a sense-making device, not only in relation to the symptoms it organizes, but also in relation to the life that it potentially curtails.

Carel also turns to Epicurus, whose philosophy is different from Heidegger's but also directed towards the problem of approaching death with tranquillity, or as he calls it, *ataraxia*. He believes that we should worry only about things we experience, and we cannot experience death. An individual might worry about dying, and associated suffering, but that is a different state of affairs. We will either suffer briefly, in which case, it's not such a big deal; it will cease. Or we will suffer chronically, a state to which we can adapt.

Epicurus maintains that happiness comes from things for which we have the capacity within ourselves. The more we find happiness from our own self-sufficiency, such as in friendship and in relinquishing the fear of death, we become located in the "here and now, cherishing the present and not being preoccupied by plans and projects."[38]

Epicurus thought of philosophy as "medicine for the soul,"[39] and Carel uses a philosophical approach not only to make intellectual sense of the dire diagnosis that is otherwise abstract for many of us, but she has experienced first-hand, but also to provide a different means for understanding diagnosis than we generally afford it in contemporary and popular culture. She proposes philosophy as therapy. Learning to live with illness, is, she writes, "learning to be happy now, regardless of threats to our future."[40]

In her "Pink Ribbons and Public Private Parts" article, Martha Stoddard Holmes anchors her analysis of her own ovarian cancer in the study of popular culture and literature.[41] Professor of literature and writing studies at California State University, Stoddard Holmes focuses on how we come to *imagine* what it is to have a particular diagnosis. She was diagnosed with ovarian cancer after seeing her GP, feeling guilty about not having had a check-up in a long time, and not being really sure if she had something wrong with her or not. Stoddard Holmes's doctor palpated her abdomen as part of the check-up, felt something that she didn't believe should be there, and sent Stoddard Holmes for emergency diagnostic imaging, which located two large tumours. As Stoddard Holmes relates the story of this diagnostic journey, she ponders that even as she narrates this diagnostic episode, she is telling a story in retrospect. The diagnosis allows her to look backwards and re-instil events and sensations pre-diagnosis with diagnostic portent. At the time, they were just messy things that were there but not important. They got better, or they were weird, but with the diagnostic moment came Stoddard Holmes's capacity to link them, make them cohere, explain their oddities.

But what if she had been able to make sense of this earlier? she muses. She knew there was something interesting in her abdomen. To read her account, however, it would appear that she didn't think of it as potentially life-threatening. What is ovarian cancer after all? How would it be part of the consciousness of any given woman? These organs, so deeply hidden in a woman's body, and usually only considered in the context of childbearing and menstruation, disappear in public and individual consciousness. These are not the breasts with which we are obsessed, which are part of a pink ribbon campaign and celebrity revelations. As Stoddard Holmes writes, "few of us ever imagine or actively experience the ovaries at all unless we have a compelling reason to do so."[42] She adds she had no idea of their size, "nor could [she] locate them unless a medical professional was palpating them."[43]

Stoddard Holmes's intellectual documentary is one in which she explores the popular rhetoric of organs and diagnosis and its role in creating a public imaginary. Diagnoses that are seen as "silent" or "symptomless" may actually be diseases for which individuals have no means of imagining. To think about what's happening inside our bodies we need, she explains, a "triangulation" between our sensations and a news report, a film, or a public health campaign. It is being able to imagine these sensations into the concrete diagnostic category that compels us to seek medical attention and take steps towards treatment.

As a scholar of popular culture, Stoddard Holmes invites her readers to consider the "artefacts" of diagnosis: visual cues, symbols, clinical signs. The pink ribbon of the breast cancer awareness campaign gives "the public a way to picture cancer without actually picturing cancer – or even a way to actively *non-think* cancer – the ribbons and bracelets may effectively neutralize the stigma of the person with cancer and return him or her to the human circle."[44]

But what of ovarian cancer, this disease so hard to imagine by virtue of its location and its inconspicuousness? What is its place in popular culture? Stoddard Holmes reminds us (if we ever even knew) the names of some prominent individuals who were diagnosed with ovarian cancer: Coretta Scott King, Gilda Radner, and Laura Nyro, she tells us. She highlights the memoir of Liz Tilberis (*No Time to Die: Living with Ovarian Cancer*). Stoddard Holmes brings to our attention the National Ovarian Cancer Coalition's Walk for the Whisper and its teal ribbon (which hasn't retained the same impact as the pink one of breast cancer). She points out ovarian cancer in *Wit* (see our discussion of this in chapter 5) in the television show *Thirtysomething* and in one episode of *Grey's Anatomy*, and in Richard Powers's novel *Gain*.

There are therefore some public narratives about ovarian cancer but not many. That there are so few cannot be explained, maintains Stoddard Holmes, by the relative incidence of ovarian cancer in relation to, for example, breast cancer. After all, ovarian cancer is the fifth cause of cancer deaths among women. Stoddard Holmes reflects on historical and cultural approaches to gender and to women's health and proposes that ovarian cancer "acts as an intensification and focalization of a superpathological site inside the already diseased female body."[45] As Fleischmann had suggested in her own essay, like any other body part, the ovaries carry culturally determined meaning, in this case, perhaps of the hysterical woman, always potentially ill (see Patricia Vertinsky's "The Eternally Wounded Woman,"[46] which reveals how menstruation was historically cast as rendering Victorian women lesser-than and more feeble than men).

Stoddard Holmes's work illustrates the incredible importance of the discourses available to the general public to make sense of the precursor symptoms of potentially serious diseases. While on the one hand her work could be made mandatory reading in Public Health 101, it also serves another important function. When we have fear or deliver (in the case of clinicians) particular diagnoses, we would do well to devote time to understanding their popular representation as much as their pathophysiological or epidemiological meaning. To have, or to deliver, a diagnosis requires the capacity to imagine what is going on, and that imagination is grounded in popular culture.

———

There are, of course, many other powerful illness narratives, while in the absence of methodological approach for understanding the diagnosis, still paint rich accounts of the diagnosis and its impact. Audré Lorde's *The Cancer Journals* was originally published in 1980. In the pages of this book, the renowned poet, feminist, lesbian, and activist wrote of her experience of breast cancer diagnosis and mastectomy. She wrote that "feelings need voice, in order to be recognized, respected and of use"[47] and to overcome the "commonality of isolation and painful reassessment which is shared by all women with breast cancer."[48] Her story of diagnosis is one of community and solidarity. She woke up from general anaesthesia after a biopsy, aware, as she put her hands to her chest, that the surgeon must have found cancer. Her doctor had said he would biopsy both breasts if he found a malignancy in one; she could feel the dressings on both breasts. It was a giveaway. "It is malignant, isn't it, Frances, it is malignant," she queried her lover.

Art Frank calls Lorde's narrative one of resistance. It is shaped by who Lorde is, by her affiliations, her identity. That she is African-American, queer, and female gives voice to different possibilities in the diagnosis story. It gives a "horizon ... within which aspects of the world are selected for attention, and what is selected is evaluated"[49] even though she draws, nonetheless, on pre-existing narrative resources: authentic though her account might be, no illness narrative, Frank argues, is ever strictly individual.[50]

Rita Charon explains that narratives demonstrate "how critical is the telling of pain and suffering, enabling patients to give voice to what they endure and to frame the illness so as to escape dominion by it."[51] The healing process begins with the narrative, she writes, "when patients tell of symptoms or even fears of illness – first to themselves, then to loved ones, and finally to health professionals."[52] Charon contextualizes these views in relation to narrative medicine, an approach to medical education and practice that explores the importance of listening to, and telling stories, as a way to promote effective health outcomes. Her words above highlight how understanding narratives contribute to the practice of medicine: being able to identify the context of illness, beliefs about causality, characters, and emotions contribute to understanding what a patient is experiencing. It aids the doctors to recognize both their patients' and their own singularity in among the generalizing grasp of the diagnosis, the algorithm, and the protocol: "Using narrative knowledge enables a person [to] understand the plight of another by participating in his or her story with complex skills of imagination, interpretation, and recognition," she underlines.[53]

The narratives discussed above go beyond the individual stories of the diagnosed women to offer techniques for understanding them. While based in singularity, each one of these authors looked for the general and did so via their disciplinary expertise.

As I started to pull together this book, and considered what it should include, it seemed to me that the most important thing it could offer my readers would be a different way of looking at a phenomenon for which most of us already have a conceptual model. At the start of this chapter, I described how stories, too, could be told *differently* highlighting the helpful, rather than the destructive, powers of diagnosis. The problem with the models we use, the stories we tell, is that we rarely have any distance from, or a critical sense of, how we've arrived upon them or what other ways we might have for looking at or narrating a problem. We resort easily to tropes and prominent templates

I am, myself, a sociologist and tend to look at problems through a sociological lens, which is concerned with structures and values and where power resides in any particular conflict or enigma. But at the same time, I work as a health professional, and I use a very different perspective to consider problems when I arrive on the scene of an emergency in my community (I work as a rural first responder for the ambulance service). While I rely on clinical reasoning when I decide what steps to take with my patient, having access to sociological tools may be far more powerful as I debrief with the emergency rescue team after the event. Why did things work (or not!) as we expected?

Sociologists Glaser and Strauss commented on the potential of having different disciplinary points of view for making sense of phenomena. Of course, they considered sociology a helpful alternative to clinicians: "The most useful sociological accounts are precisely those which insiders recognize as sufficiently inside to be true but not so 'inside' that they reveal only what is already known ... The sociologist's obligation is to report honestly but according to his own lights," they wrote.[54] My reading of this is that the account of the sociologist is one which will *resonate* with the clinician; the clinician herself could not have constructed this particular account without the sociologist's (different) ways of analysing the phenomenon.

What this says is that the sociologist is in a privileged position, with access to a different set of tools and theoretical and epistemological foundations for examining the challenges faced by Western medicine, its practitioners, and those who seek its support. The sociology of diagnosis, understood in the terms of Glaser and Strauss, provides a critical perspective of the practice of medicine, viewing its limitations and constraints from outside of the values which engender it, and acknowledging the power dynamics at play in the practice of medicine.

But sociology alone is not enough. Or perhaps I should say, classic sociology is not enough. I have previously written about what I call multi-contextual critical diagnostic studies.[55] My thinking about situating sociology in a much broader context comes from the writings of sociologist Eviatar Zerubavel, whom I mentioned in chapter 4. His approach is to study social problems across context, media, and era to uncover what he refers to as enduring social "patterns."[56] Zerubavel's social pattern analysis is an approach inspired by Simmel, which seeks to understand a social structure or phenomenon by studying it as broadly as possible, across as many contexts as possible. Social pattern analysis is indifferent to "singularity," or to what appear unique and discrete instantiations of particular behaviours. Rather, in social pattern analysis, one is "purposely oblivious to the idiosyncratic features of the communities, events or situations that they study, looking for general patterns that transcend their specific instantiations."[57] The comparisons that emerge from social pattern analysis are designed to "highlight the formal commonality rather than the cultural, historical or situational singularity of the various specific manifestations of that pattern."[58]

The diagnostic process is remarkably well suited to the trans-everything approach Zerubavel describes. In fact, ideas about diagnosis only make sense within a wider structure of thought. When the sociologist considers the spectrum of ways in which diagnosis is illustrated, it is clear that situating the study of diagnosis in a wide context opens up the subject to the multiple viewing perspectives from which diagnosis is identified, promoted, enacted and experienced. To overlook creative interpretation of diagnosis (film, theatre, poetry, fiction), for example, is to shut off potential symbolic meanings poignantly understood by viewers/readers and potentially more powerful in understanding the social dynamics of the diagnostic moment as is a qualitative observational study. Similarly, the use of cultural and historical data provides rich sources in the pursuit of commonality, "compar[ing] phenomena that may be radically different in concrete content yet essentially similar in structural arrangement."[59] This follows Douglas who wrote: "the right basis for comparison is to insist on the unity of human experience and at the same time to insist on its variety and the differences which make comparison worthwhile."[60]

So, as I assembled these "intellectual documentaries," I was curious about what these linguistic, philosophical, literary, and also sociological interpretations would offer. Convinced of the important contribution such different approaches would make to my readers, I was also aware of my own disciplinary anchors. Would an Epicurean or a semantic analysis of the diagnosis resonate with me, as Glaser and Strauss maintained a sociological analysis should with a similar outsider?

These essays strike many chords. They were familiar yet novel: perspectives I couldn't might not have easily uncovered from my own disciplinary vantage point. I am reminded, for example, of how one of my sisters refers to her physical ailments. Instead of explaining that her arthritic knee is sore, she'll more likely explain that "her knee is not happy" or that "her knee is bothering her" or even that "her knee is doing what it does." By using this syntactical construction, I can now see, she is likely distancing herself, perhaps from this thing that she has not found a way to overcome. She is making her arthritis external to herself and to her volition. At the same time, I can also see the potential risks in linguistically constructing diagnostic description in one way as opposed to another, because of the very same or similar semantic consequences.

I can also see how so many diseases are linguistically constructed in general terms before they unleash any personal impact. Have you noticed that people who die from cancer are often referred to as *victims*, as if cancer had some particular agency and intent to attack? We may *fall victim* to the cold, fire, heat (or to violence!), but with the exception of cancer, we aren't usually referred to as *falling victim* to many other diseases. Even if we are undiagnosed, and are not ill or diseased, that we would think of cancer as something lurking in the background ready to *victimize* us pre-shapes the cancer we or our associates may one day experience.

There is no doubt that these authors, in writing the stories of their own diagnoses, accomplished the same thing as they might have were they writing a generic illness narrative. In each of these essays, there is a clear personal engagement with illness and, more importantly (for the purposes of this book), with a diagnosis. But there is also an attempt to achieve something generic in their personal narrative. By exploring their phenomenological experience of diagnosis with their disciplinary overlays, they provide different ways of explaining, studying, and improving the diagnostic process and its announcement.

They are not alone in writing such accounts. Art Frank, to whom I referred to previously in this book (and this chapter) has been writing about the illness experience from a sociological and humanistic approach for over 20 years. But so too have Ann Oakley,[61] Elizabeth Ettorre,[62] PJ Caplan,[63] or even poet Raymond Carver,[64] whose "What the Doctor Said" distils powerfully the impact of a lung cancer diagnosis, by describing how he thanked the doctor for his diagnosis, "habit being so strong."

To understand any subject critically requires a multifaceted and multi-epistemic approach to the subject. By *multi-epistemic* I mean coming from different sources of knowledge. There is not one absolute way to understand the "truth" of a subject. That I put the word *truth* in emphatic quotation marks is precisely to underline that truth is not a fixed entity; there are many ways of knowing truth. Readers of this book about stories are likely easy to convince that, for example, statistics and numbers convey only part of the truth of diagnosis. But, even if they are sociologists, like I, they might not have considered the many other ways of thinking sociologically about diagnosis. These authors provide us with a range of approaches that reveal more than we could reveal on our own, with the tools we normally hold in our hands. They expand our thinking about how diagnosis and diagnoses operate and frame our sense of the world, of health, and of illness. To have a true critical understanding of diagnosis, we must look at various disciplinary locations to explore the full impact of diagnosis as an object of study.

CHAPTER EIGHT

What's There to Tell?
Diagnosis-as-Mystery

I started this book claiming that diagnostic stories were prevalent, influential, and invisible. I proposed to reveal their presence and describe the way in which they exerted various forms of power to reassemble these narratives in ways that might dilute their dominant impact. As I come to the end of this book, I propose one last diagnostic narrative and highlight its alternative potential.

One rainy evening, I happened to catch a glimpse of *The Avengers*. This 2012 production by Joss Whedon is a live-action version of the Marvel comic strip by the same name, first produced in the early 1960s. The story is about a team of superheroes, ever vigilant to save the world and its people from external forces. Hulk, Captain America, Iron Man, Thor, and others fight "the foes no single superhero can withstand."[1]

I arrived in time to see on the screen a handsome and well-built naked man (actor Mark Ruffalo) in a pile of rubble, not-quite-modestly concealed by bits of cinder block.

"Who's that?" I pestered the children who were clustered around the television.

"That's Hulk!" they replied in gleeful unison

I settled in to watch. A security guard appeared on the screen, looking down at the naked Hulk who appeared dazed, trying to make sense of where he was.

"Did I hurt anybody?" asks Hulk with a blurred tongue.

"There's nobody 'round here to get hurt" replies the guard, played by actor Harry Dean Stanton. "You did scare the hell out of some pigeons though."

"Lucky!"
     "Or just good aim. You were awake when you fell."
     "You saw?"
     "The whole thing! You went through the ceiling. Big and green and buck-ass nude. Here [throws some clothes at Hulk]. I didn't think these would fit you until you shrunk down to a regular-sized feller."
     "Thank you."
     "Are you an alien?"
     "What ... ?"
     "From outer space? An alien [enunciating carefully]."
     "Nah."
     "Well then, son. *You've* got a condition."[2]

This interesting scene was both similar to and different from many of the diagnostic narratives I've presented thus far. Like others, the diagnosis was used to make sense of the social world and the action of its characters. In this case, the diagnosis (even though the diagnosis was pretty basic – "a condition" – and the person proclaiming the diagnosis was not a doctor) was a way of communicating between Hulk, the security guard, and the viewers that something wasn't quite right about Hulk (see figure 8.1). It was explanatory, pulling together a range of phenomena, linking them, and giving a rationale for their presence. The *differential diagnosis*[3] was unusual, of course, "alien" versus "condition." It served an important place in the plot, giving Banner some sort of framework via which he could accept his superhuman powers.[4]

But this scene did something very different as well. For Banner, being told he had a "condition," even if only by a janitor, was not a moment of transformation. It was a simple observation of fact and fate. It was something that needed to be taken in stride, not something that disruptive. The destabilizing power was outside of the diagnostic moment. "Having a condition" was obvious and matter of fact. The power of naming, however, was disarmed by telling the story in terms other than of transformation. Banner was not distressed by being told something was seriously wrong with him. He just nods, grunts, and starts to get dressed.

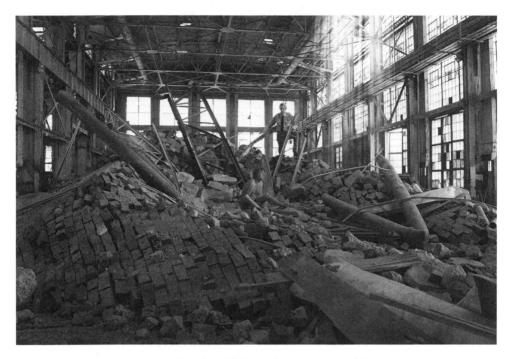

8.1 Bruce Banner (Mark Ruffalo) and security guard (Harry Dean
Stanton), in *The Avengers*: Is the Hulk an alien, or does he
have a "condition"?

This diagnostic scene counters the tendency in contemporary narrative constructions, be they about diagnosis or something else, to focus
on personal change. It is a trend that novelist Damien Wilkins laments,
as it "leaves out other ways of being in the world." It's not that transformation stories don't have their place, but there are other ways of
telling stories. Save the powerful about-turns for when they matter, he
argues: "The notion of personal change – change which is improving –
is both disreputable and unmoveable, tarnished and resolute, art's
cheapest trick and its most generous gift."[5] Narratives don't always
have to promise change. If we hearken back to the Greeks, the dominant narrative form focused on observing what happened to people as
they endured trials. The trials were administered by fate, and rather
than *transforming* the characters, they *revealed* them. They ride on, and
through, the chaos of life, with only fate as immovable. In contrast to

the change narrative (like the one I propose in the Introduction at the moment the doctor is going to tell us the name of some dreaded malady), it is not a moment where a power structure is revealed. The narrative affirms rather than changes the character.[6]

Wilkins proposes that the personality "as mystery" rather than "as transformed" communicates powerful messages in narrative, and turns to "reliable hindsight" to deliver its import. Transformation is not the only tale worth telling. Building upon Wilkins's musings, I see a clear appeal in the idea of considering *diagnosis-as-mystery* rather than *as truth*. While the diagnostic moment is one in which information is exchanged, laboratory values explained, and prognoses considered, it is not a moment of truth and need not be a moment of transformation.

Diagnosis is not a moment of transformation for Superman, in the *All-Star Superman* scene I described earlier. Superman's diagnosis of irreversible cellular apoptosis is actually the consequence of his heroism. As he saved the Earth from deadly stellar radiation, he absorbed such levels of radiation himself that he now suffers from cell death. His death is certain and proximate. Ironically, in this series, which is based on superhuman transformation, the diagnostic moment is quite blasé. Superman takes a moment and stares out into the world vacantly. "there are ... *things* I have to do first," he finally replies, as he goes off on another rescue.[7] He makes no further reference to his apoptosis in the volume, although he does occasionally think about his impending death with wonderment.

Audré Lorde takes a similar stance in *The Cancer Journals*: "Every once in a while I would think ... 'how do I act to announce or preserve my new status as temporary upon this earth?' and then I'd remember that we have always been temporary, and that I had just never really underlined it before, or acted out of it so completely before. And then I would feel a little foolish and needlessly melodramatic, but only a little,"[8] ... "for once we accept the actual existence of our dying, who can ever have power over us again?"[9]

I return to that question of truth-telling, linked to the diagnostic moment. It's one that physicians find difficult to tussle with. Not surprising, of course, if we look at the stories of chapter 3; the medical edifice is built on this configuration. This is more than just an academic affair. Why we should consider diagnosis to be about "truth" as opposed to, say, information or explanation, is an important matter to ponder in practice. When I have presented to medical audiences and asked doctors to consider thinking about telling a patient her diagnosis in terms

other than that of "truth-telling" I am usually met with the protesta-
tion "But it is true! What do you want us to call it ... lies?" This is a
false dichotomy. Stating that you are hungry, my name is Annemarie,
and there is traffic on the motorway is true, but uninteresting in that
capacity. These facts, as they are – and as is a diagnosis – are interesting in their sense-making, not in their truth. And referring to them as
"truths" reinforces the power differential between patient and doctor.
Allan Barry posits that it is precisely the power differential that creates "truth." He explains the "differences between true and false do
not exist apart from the practice in which these values are produced
and evaluated and statements made to circulate as true, as known or
probable ... the practice conditions situate truth amid the major asym-
metries of social power, undermining its status as common good."[10]

It is not truth that counts as much as the implications of the information, the links that it creates with treatments and outcomes, the way in
which it enables the self.[11] But it is by couching diagnosis in terms of
truth that pushes its function away from sense-making to wholesale
transformation. Who holds the keys to the truth then controls the discourse, adds weight to its assertions, and controls the models by which
health, illness, and disease are understood.[12]

As I have demonstrated throughout the book, diagnosis is a powerful
tool in the telling of stories. It triggers them, it shapes them, it invents
them. Recall Stoddard Holmes's story of her ovarian cancer. She told
a story that was untellable before her diagnosis. The diagnosis drew
together the events that otherwise bore no relationship to one another
without the unifying potential of, in this case, ovarian cancer.

In this final chapter, I want to turn to how all of these readings of
diagnostic narratives matter in the practical arenas of health and the
provision of health care. Let me tell another story. One of my grand-
sons has serious asthma. He has regular stints in the hospital and three
different-coloured puffers in his little medicine bag. While I was working on this manuscript, I had just received a copy of Ian Williams's *The
Bad Doctor*[13] and I had left it on the table in the dining room. Ian drew/
wrote the graphic diagnosis chapter in this *Diagnosis: Truths and Tales*.
My grandson walked by and picked up the book, intrigued by the cartoon drawings.

"The Bad Doctor," he deciphered carefully. "Why is the doctor bad?"
he asked, curious. He was enthralled by the pictures of stethoscopes,
nurses, and doctors with which he was so familiar, but he was too young
to understand the metaphysical angst with which Dr Iwan James was

dealing in Ian's graphic novel. I went to the graphic medicine website to see if I could find something better suited to a six-year-old child.

I found a comic called *Iggy and the Inhalers* online. I opened it up in its online version to show my grandson. *Iggy and the Inhalers* is a cartoon about asthma that was designed as an educational tool for children and uses the superhero genre to make the inhalers and the health threats livelier and more enthralling for the children it is targeting as its readership.[14]

"This is about asthma," I started to explain.

"What's asthma?" he asked. And then the penny dropped. This little boy didn't know that he had a diagnosis. He knew when he was sick, and he knew what that sickness entailed, but he didn't have a name for this sickness. Without a diagnosis, he could still take his puffers and still understand that he was sick, but as we read through the cartoon together, I became aware that children, like adults, become *socialized* to diagnosis. And that socialization serves an important purpose.

My grandson grabbed on to the concept of diagnosis with great interest. It organized his symptoms and treatment in the way that Balint described in 1964, even though with a child, there was no negotiation involved. He is now able to explain bronchial inflammation and the role of the preventer (Coltron the Controller) and the reliever (Broncho the Bronchodilator) as if they were characters in *The Avengers*.

The proponents of graphic medicine would say "Aha!" and use this as an example of how the graphic medium can bridge the gap between clinical knowledge and personal experience of disease. Cartoons can become an effective intervention for patient education and disease awareness. The stories they tell are sometimes easier to assimilate than more traditional written pamphlets.

But that's not what is happening in *The Avengers*. With no educational intent, it nonetheless educated. The story of the more-than-human Banner/ Hulk reinforces what is already imprinted upon the viewers: a diagnosis explains a lot of weird stuff. A social theorist might question the diagnostic instinct. Must we diagnose all the variations of human behaviour? Isn't there some space for just accepting people as they are?

Well, clearly not when the condition makes us suffer. As grownups, we'd be hard pressed to imagine health care without diagnosis. How would we talk about what ails us in a way that our listeners would understand? Would we have to explain our fever, muscle aches, fatigue, and runny nose each time we had the flu? How would we anticipate the healing time from our mountain bike accidents without knowing whether we had a fracture of a rib or a simple bruise? Each time we'd go to the doctor, we would be seen as an individual case. Not so bad, you might think, except that it would keep the doctor from being able to apply a therapy that worked well for another case of the same thing, because we wouldn't have a way of identifying illnesses as the same without the diagnosis.

Maybe it helps, as a rule, to see a diagnosis as a story. I started this book by describing diagnosis as a narrative in and of itself. The diagnosis becomes *a story that links in a series of facts or phenomena, and explains their relationship.* Howard Brody encourages diagnosticians to think of the diagnostic process in terms of storytelling. His article entitled "My Story Is Broken; Can You Help Me Fix It?" describes how the encounter between patient and doctor with a diagnostic aim is actually an opportunity for a jointly constructed narrative in which patients makes themselves known via their stories, and the diagnostician both receives and accepts patients' stories to relieve suffering:

> The physician who hopes to heal and to relieve suffering ought to attend as seriously to the patient's story of the illness experience as to the purely bodily manifestations of disease. (Put more accurately, the physician should approach a deeper inquiry into bodily processes through the vehicle of the patient's story.) And the physician should approach the story in a way that encourages the ultimate goal of shared power: making the patient a more active participant in his medical care.[15]

Brody explains that during co-construction, patients must be convinced that the proposed narrative is about their case and not a stock-standard story that the doctor takes off the shelf and hands out to all. The co-constructed narrative resembles Balint's negotiation model and is a strong cornerstone to the narrative medicine movement.[16]

Before I say more about narrative medicine, I return to the idea of the boundary object. I started this book by talking about the ways in which diagnostic stories are a disciplinary boundary object. A common item of interest for many disciplines, each having a different variant on what theoretical tack will allow us to comprehend its function, the narratives of diagnosis sit at the heart of an imaginary Venn diagram. I underline the s in *narratives* to highlight the multiplicity of narratives that converge for each diagnostic moment (patient, doctor, family, popular culture, and so on). Narratives are inescapable, complex, and multifaceted. These complex diagnostic narratives are also boundary objects in practice.

The practice to which I refer is clinical, creative, personal, intellectual, and more. Narrative medicine is one example, but there are many more. A script writer might choose to make her character cough, later taking him to the doctor's office to find out what is wrong. She does it for a reason. A doctor listens carefully to a patient's story of a candidate diagnosis to try to figure out how his own medical knowledge can be used as a sense-making tool … or not. Diagnosis stories intersect and serve different purposes within their intersecting places of practice.

Narrative medicine, as one place of practice, is concerned with how patients narrate their experiences of illness, how understanding the stories in medical case history can help support clinical care, and how narrative can be used as a treatment modality.[17] Understanding the operation of narratives helps the clinician to make more sense of the patient's accounts, postures, means of storytelling, and self-awareness. It promotes responsiveness to the different power relations and epistemologies in the diagnostic setting.[18] Charon subtitles one of her chapters "To Profess Is a Narrative Act" and describes narrative as bringing the profession together, bridging differences, and promoting patient interests.[19] I concur, although I will add to her argument that narrative competency must pay attention to diagnostic tropes. The patient narrative as a means of establishing the personal context of disease does not fulfil its potential if the diagnosis comes in, cookie-cutter style, to impose a tired and conventional transformation.

Another practice setting is narrative therapy. In a narrative approach to psychotherapy and social work, the client recasts his or her story of identity through a guided retelling.[20] In bibliotherapy, on the other hand, healing is promoted by reading stories, along with, frequently, writing therapy. Using stories to heal is not a recent affair. The Egyptian pharaoh Ramses the Great is said to have had the inscription "the house of healing for the soul" inscribed above the door of his library.[21] Much more recently, a Dr Johnson discussed the "prescription of literature" as an important therapeutic. He quoted Gerald Webb's who believed that "there are many times when it is incumbent on the wise physician to prescribe, not a posset or a purgative, but an essay or a poem," explaining how caring for patients involves, above all, caring for their mental state, for which "the right kind of literature" is an effective remedy.[22] Librarian Clifton McAlistair in the *American Journal of Nursing* also proclaimed. "A library in a psychiatric hospital should be considered as a prescription unit!" and recommended that the nurse work with the librarian to obtain the best effect for the patients.[23]

But in line with the "Intellectual Documentaries" of the previous chapter, and with the sociological tradition where I have based my scholarship, I am less interested in the micro-level use of narrative in the doctor-patient encounter than I am in the cultural setting in which we tell diagnostic stories. In this book, I have shown how diagnosis stories are everywhere we turn, on television, in the theatre, in our newspapers and novels, and indeed in (but most importantly, outside of) our doctors' offices. But they are not just pervasive, they are persuasive. Whether or not it is their intent (and most frequently, it is not), they cast a particular view of diagnosis and its transformative potential. They locate power in particular arenas, and awareness of the location of power allows teller and listener to reposition it.

It behoves any clinician (and indeed, readers of this book, interested as they must be, in disease and diagnosis from some perspective, to have made it to this last chapter) to be alert to these culturally-prevalent stories. As we diagnose, or are diagnosed with, any particular disorder, the sense we make of it will be shaped by the cultural models on offer. As Stoddard Holmes explained in her "Pink Ribbons" essay, we have ways of imaging our insides, and the diseases that afflict us. How we imagine these things depends on what popular configurations are available to us.

She relies on the work of Damasio to explain how the feelings we experience in our own bodies are narrativized by external depictions:

> The foundational images in the stream of mind are images of some kind of body event, whether the event happens in the depth of the body or in some specialized sensory device near its periphery. The basis for those foundational images is a collection of brain maps [that] ... represent, comprehensively, the structure and state of the body at any given time. (Damasio in Stoddard Holmes, p. 478)

She focuses on the public images, texts, information, and narratives about diagnosis which pervade our experience of contemporary society. Stoddard Holmes, despite her academic location in literary criticism, leans towards the medical humanities *for* medicine, commenting on how the absence of representation of her diagnosis in popular culture affected her understanding of the "facts" of disease, but in so doing, she gives weight to a point that Frank makes about the illness narrative from the perspective of medical *critique*. In every story of diagnosis, he explains, we are always co-creating, always drawing on pre-existing narrative motifs, always leaning upon existing communities of expression, of diagnosis.[24] This is yet another example of why the critical recognition of what these motifs impose and what other manners we have for narrating diagnosis are so important.

Notably, there is also room to consider what motifs are absent and salience of their absence. There are here matters of class and of heteronormativity that are captured in the dominant diagnostic narrative motifs, and which, with only a few exceptions (notably, films like *Bíutiful* and authors like Audré Lorde) leave numerous models for experience illness and the medical encounter unexplored. Narratives of diagnosis often resemble the one with which I opened this book, in which the narrator (me) comes from a comfortable middle class where she can expect to consult a doctor and is likely to be welcomed, or at least allowed, into the medical realm to the degree that such is possible for a non-doctor.

Whether teller, listener, or watcher of diagnostic moments, we can consider how our engagement with the diagnosis in its many narrative guises prompts us to imagine our diagnosticians and even ourselves in the diagnostic process. Do we think about dementia the way it is depicted in *Still Alice*, with a family reshaping and conforming itself to a new reality? Will we, in the same dignified and graceful way as Alice did, inform our employers, self-monitor our ability to deliver lectures to the masses, stepping down at the propitious time? Will we relinquish ourselves to our offspring, offering, in a kind of trade, our self-actualization in exchange for theirs? Or do we think about dementia the way it is represented in *Da Vinci's Inquest*, with an identity-less walker, cut off from civilized society, and left to roam the public park?[25]

How also do these representations shape our expectations of the diagnosticians we approach to help us make sense of our dysfunctions? From the deathless man in *The Tiger's Wife*[26] to *House, MD*[27] and *Wit*,[28] we have an array of different models to choose from: the doctor as demon, as detective, or as adversary. Oh, and let's not forget the marvellous caring doctor, our friend, whom we hope will come to our rescue as in *The Various Haunts of Man*[29] or *A Late Quartet*,[30] and who serves as the ideal in most of the medical writings featured in *Diagnosis: Truths and Tales*.

Whether we imagine our doctors as detectives who will be able to sort the wheat from the chaff and – presto! – uncover the truth of our suffering or as condescending power mongers, like the antagonist in *Wit*, it is the stories that circulate about doctors that will help elucidate the ways in which people anticipate what they will achieve by consulting a physician, and from what departure point they will start to tell their own tale of illness or of health. As Blaxter reminded us, it is important to see structures above simple communication.[31] We are never looking at just one person's story. We are always looking at a story which emerges from a tradition of stories.

But sometimes stories, like common sense, are based on assumptions that clearly need crucial, critical reconsideration and can be retold together. Have you ever returned to a book you loved when you were a teenager? Have you, with a bit of distance, seen new themes and moralistic messages that weren't apparent to you as a child? I have just finished reading Madeleine L'Engle's *Wrinkle in Time*.[32] What to me was a science fiction adventure as a 12-year-old is today a plea to young adults to accept themselves as they are and not necessarily in the image of their peers, and to see love, loyalty, and justice as the important values that will serve them throughout life.

Re-viewing *House, MD*, or *Grey's Anatomy* (the least subtle of the diagnosis stories) with a bit of distance (hopefully, reading *Diagnosis: Truths and Tales* provides some critical tools for so doing) reveals different stories than the initial viewing might have: that diagnostic authority instils the diagnostician with power, that diagnosis is a device of characterization, that diagnosis is cast as forensic in nature. We might not have thought about these options as we snort with disbelief when one of the members of House's retinue proposes, yet again, "It could be sarcoidosis" (it seems like every time the team was stumped, they suggest either lupus or sarcoidosis, both rather non-specific, systemic autoimmune illnesses).

At the same time, if we were watching the show from the personal perspective of a diagnosis of lupus or sarcoidosis, we might not snort, but turn away in despair. Why is the disease by which we are affected so regularly used as a kind of symbolic wastebasket diagnosis that looks like everything and at the same time like nothing? Does it mean that people by extension snort with disbelief when we give them the diagnostic explanation for our illness? "Sarcoidosis? You've gotta be kidding! Like on *House*?"

As we are reminded by H. Porter Abbott in his *Cambridge Introduction to Narrative*, "Narrative often is, an instrument that provokes active thinking and helps us work through problems, even as we tell about them or hear them being told. But ... it is also important to note that narrative can be used to deliver false information; it can be used to keep us in darkness and even encourage us to do things we should not do. This too must be kept in mind."[33]

As I draw this book to a close, Abbott's points give me important ways of pulling all of these musings about diagnosis and its narratives together. He underlines the important organizational and explanatory potential of narrative, while simultaneously pointing out its limitation as a device for making sense of, in the present case, illness. With this in mind, we need to keep telling, listening to, and challenging stories. The "narrative templates" that shape the profound experience of health and illness provide us with strength and insight, as much as with trepidation. As we tell and listen to our own stories in our heads, or the stories that are handed to us, we can cherish them as stories and value the potential they offer us, but also consider that on any one subject, or any specific presentation, there are many other possible stories to tell.

It is not enough to say that films and fiction aren't real and that we must dispel the myths created by popular culture. The accuracy of the stories in popular texts is not the point, rather it is their function – the values they embody the qualities they promote, the roles of their characters, the thinking they provoke – which matter in the evaluation of narratives. Knowing this enables the creation of new narratives, just as satisfying, and probably more useful, both personally and clinically.

Notes

Introduction

1 Schofield, *Unconscious Therapeutics*.
2 Leder, *The Absent Body*.
3 Fleischman, "A Linguist Reflects."
4 Lacey, *Image and Representation*.
5 Star and Griesemer, "Institutional Ecology."
6 Star and Griesemer, 411.
7 Star and Griesemer, 412.
8 Latour, "Why Has Critique Run out of Steam?"
9 Charon and Montello, *Stories Matter*.
10 For example, Boesky, *The Story Within*; De Shazer and Helle, "Theorizing Breast Cancer."
11 For example, Gelsomini et al., "Wildcard"; Houston et al., "African American Veterans Storytelling"; and Tielman et al., "A Therapy System for Post-Traumatic Stress Disorder."
12 Klawiter, "Breast Cancer in Two Regimes."
13 Hunsaker Hawkins, "Pathography."
14 Arnold, *On the Divisions and Mutual Relations of Knowledge*.
15 Arnold, x.
16 Plato, *Plato in Twelve Volumes*, 535.
17 Willis, *The Remaining Medical Works*.
18 Lemon, *English Etymology*.

19 Blaxter, "Diagnosis as Category and Process."
20 Hacking, "Inaugural Lecture," 7.
21 Aronowitz, "Framing Disease," 1.
22 For more on this, read Stearns, *Fat History*; Jutel, "The Emergence of Overweight."
23 This judgment is just as much about the doctor as it is about the patient. The ability to diagnose correctly is also a moment in which their clinical nous is presented, where mistakes can be made, where diagnostic, but also communication, skills are highlighted.
24 Just being able to access medical records is a complex and highly structured event. Usually a series of permissions are needed. Institutions frequently prevent patients from having access in case the perspective held by the patient and the doctor are at odds and may present interpretive risks to one or the other. Ian Williams's graphic chapter (chapter 6) underlines this particular problem.
25 Frank, "Just Listening."
26 Locock et al., "'I Knew before I Was Told'"; Blaxter, "Life Narratives."
27 Davison, Smith, and Frankel, "Lay Epidemiology and the Prevention Paradox."
28 Fludernik, *Towards a "Natural" Narratology*.
29 Nor, of course, is it necessarily a positive experience. Certain labels may impose a stigma like indelible ink. Again, see Ian Williams's graphic chapter for an example.
30 Bowker and Star, *Sorting Things Out*.
31 See, for example, Wailoo, *Drawing Blood*; Metzl, *The Protest Psychosis*.
32 Parsons, "Definitions of Health and Illness."
33 Fadiman, *The Spirit Catches You*.
34 Davison, Smith, and Frankel, "Lay Epidemiology and the Prevention Paradox."
35 Johnson, *The True Physician*, 146–7.
36 Mitchell, *Conduct of the Medical Life*, 24–5.
37 Schuster, "Personalizing Illness and Modernity." Schuster's paper does question whether Mitchell's seemingly repressive approach to Perkins Gilman might be the result of a poor doctor-patient relationship more than it was a desire to repress a woman's intellectual work. He encouraged other female neurasthenic patients to write as a form of therapy.
38 Gilman, *The Yellow Wall Paper*.
39 Charon, *Narrative Medicine*, viii.
40 Charon, 50.
41 Broyard, "Doctor, Talk to Me," 179.

42 Carel, "With Bated Breath."
43 Harrison, *Medical Ethics*, 10.
44 For example, Cathell, *The Physician Himself*, 107.
45 Stoddard Holmes, "Pink Ribbons and Public Private Parts."
46 Hippocrates, "Prognosis," 170.
47 Reiser, "Words as Scalpels."
48 Hadra, 60.
49 Morpurgo, *Alone on a Wide, Wide Sea*, 14.
50 Also the sub-title of Havi Carel's book and an Epicurean quotation about happiness.
51 Carel, *Illness*.
52 Abbott, *The Cambridge Introduction to Narrative*, 12.

1 A Touch of the Flu

1 Surbone, "Truth Telling."
2 Although, as I finished writing this manuscript, Tour de France rider George Bennet, who, after three quarters of the race, was sitting comfortably in the top 10, had just abandoned the race citing "a bad case of man-flu" (https://www.cyclingweekly.com/news/racing/tour-de-france/george-bennett-abandoning-tour-de-france-cant-describe-sucks-342664). This statement is an attempt to recast the representation of influenza. Even "real men" get the flu, Bennett is telling us. Or perhaps more pointedly, he is attempting to legitimize his illness as "real," as a valid explanation for withdrawing from the race.
3 Translation: France. Flu kills 13 residents of a rest home.
4 *Oxford English Dictionary* (2002), s.v. "Influenza, n."
5 Broughton, *Observations on the Influenza*, 7 and 8.
6 Broughton, 6 and 9.
7 Taubenberger, Hultin, and Morens, "Discovery and Characterization of the 1918 Pandemic."
8 Bresalier, "'A Most Protean Disease'"; Tognotti, "Scientific Triumphalism and Learning from Facts."
9 Potter, "A History of Influenza."
10 Potter.
11 Bowker, "The History of Information Infrastructures."
12 McNeil, "The Ethics of Hunting Down 'Patient Zero.'"
13 Nicoll, "Planning for Uncertainty."
14 Centers for Disease Control and Prevention, "Avian Influenza A."
15 Stephenson and Jamieson, "Securitising Health."

16 Nerlich and Halliday, "Avian Flu."

17 Hanne and Hawken, "Metaphors for Illness," 95.

18 Centers for Disease Control and Prevention, "Outbreak of Swine-Origin Influenza A."

19 See, for example, Wooldridge, "Swine Flu-Immigration, Death and Disease"; Judicial Watch, "Illegal Aliens Spread Swine Flu in US."

20 One News/NZPA, "New Zealand Poised for Swine Flu Results."

21 Keall, "New Zealand Added to Google Swine Flu Map."

22 Lehrer's comic song was about what countries had the nuclear bomb; not the same thing, of course, but similar in the sense that it described a competition to the bottom: https://www.youtube.com/watch?v=oRLON3ddZIw

23 Centers for Disease Control and Prevention, "Update: Novel Influenza A (H1N1) Virus Infections."

24 Epidemic and Pandemic Alert and Response, "Addressing Ethical Issues."

25 Trilla, Trilla, and Daer, "The 1918 'Spanish Flu' in Spain."

26 Trilla, Trilla, and Daer, 668.

27 World Health Organization, "WHO Issues Best Practices."

28 Jutel, "Sociology of Diagnosis"; Jutel, *Putting a Name to It*.

29 Freidson, *Profession of Medicine*, 244.

30 Jutel, "Self-Diagnosis."

31 Jutel et al., "Self-Diagnosis of Influenza." While this study took place in New Zealand, and technically we shouldn't try to generalize across nations without some kind of confirmatory study, intuitively, one senses that this would likely be the case much more broadly.

32 Hughes-Jones, "Study of Influenza," 178.

33 Prior, Evans, and Prout, "Talking about Colds and Flu."

34 Hemingway, "A Day's Wait," 19.

35 Leibmann-Smith, "Swine Flu over the Cuckoo's Nest," 31.

36 Hanne and Hawken, "Metaphors for Illness in Contemporary Media," 229.

37 Hanne and Hawken, 234.

38 Arnold, *On the Divisions and Mutual Relations of Knowledge*.

39 Budd et al. "Influenza."

40 Carrat et al., "Time Lines of Infection and Disease."

41 Jutel et al., "Self-Diagnosis of Influenza."

42 Louriz et al., "Clinical Features of the Initial Cases."

43 Jutel and Banister, "'I Was Pretty Sure I Had the Flu.'"

44 ICD Update Platform, "Influenza, Avian Flu, Flu Pandemic 2009."

45 Blaxter, "Diagnosis as Category and Process," 10.

46 Blaxter, 10.

47 Global Influenza Surveillance and Response System (GISRS), "Standard-
   ization of Terminology."

48 Bresalier, "'A Most Protean Disease,'" 484.

49 Houlihan et al., "Life Threatening Infections."

50 Shortland, "Findings of Coroner H. B. Shortland."

51 Croskerry, "Achieving Quality in Clinical Decision Making."

52 Frenkel et al., "Exceptional Patients and Communication."

53 Sachs, "Be an Optimist," 324.

54 Bettevy, Dufranc, and Hofmann, "Les enjeux du dispositif d'annonce," 517.

55 Lund, "The Doctor, the Patient and the Truth," 956.

56 Surbone, "Truth Telling," 56.

57 Rosenberg, "Contested Boundaries: Psychiatry, Disease and Diagnosis";
   Jutel, "When Pigs Could Fly."

2 Whose Stories?

1 It's not surprising that doctors refer to this part of the diagnostic process as "taking a history." There are two interesting points in labelling
   it thus. The first, of course, is the etymology of the word *history*, which
   is from the Greek *historia* or "narrative." The second is that the act of
   listening to the patient account should be described as "taking." There
   is a sense of appropriation embedded in this verb which punctuates the
   idea that diagnosis is something which is created through tension and
   control.

2 Balint, *The Doctor, His Patient and the Illness.*

3 Leder, "Clinical Interpretation."

4 Frank, *The Wounded Storyteller.*

5 Frank, 6.

6 Frank.

7 Lupton, "Consumerism, Reflexivity and the Medical Encounter."

8 The introduction of sildenafil in 1998 was characterized as the most successful market launch ever of a pharmaceutical product, with prescriptions
   of 10,000 pills per day (Hill and McKie, "Ten Years On.")

9 Lisa Rinna, an actress on the television shows *Days of Our Lives* and *Danc-
   ing with the Stars*, featured prominently on the website of the company
   initially developing one of the more promising medications (Boehringer
   Ingelheim). She reached out to everyday women, asking them to consider
   if they had the same problems as she did. See more about this in Jutel and
   Mintzes, "Female Sexual Dysfunction."

10 Balint, *The Doctor, His Patient and the Illness.* (Italics in original.)

11 Brown, "The Name Game."
12 Gualtieri, "The Doctor as the Second Opinion."
13 Krecke, *The Doctor and His Patients*, 35.
14 Anonymous, "Commerce without Conscience."
15 Gersuny, *Doctor and Patient*, 29.
16 Keith, *Clinical Case-Taking*, 16.
17 Keith, 17.
18 Lapham, *Disease and the Man*, 20.
19 Gersuny, *Doctor and Patient*, 29.
20 Hadra, *The Public and the Doctor*, 1.
21 Vorhaus, *The Changing Patient-Doctor Relationship*, 19.
22 Styrap, *A Code of Medical Ethics*, 20.
23 Gersuny, *Doctor and Patient*, 29.
24 "Mine" is in reference to the original author.
25 Bainbridge, "The Cancer Campaign Quarternary," 164.
26 Styrap, *A Code of Medical Ethics*, 25.
27 "Commerce without Conscience."
28 Brown, *Health: Five Lay Sermons to Working People*.
29 Little, *Doctors and the Public*, 8–9.
30 Brackenbury, *Patient and Doctor*, 91.
31 Te Poel et al., "The Curious Case of Cyberchondria."
32 Te Poel et al.; Doherty-Torstrick, Walton, and Fallon, "Cyberchondria: Parsing Health Anxiety from Online Behavior"; Fergus and Dolan, "Problematic Internet Use"; and Spence, "Bad Medicine."
33 Mackey, "Digital Direct-to-Consumer Advertising"; Kim, "Trouble Spots in Online Direct-to-Consumer Prescription Drug Promotion"; Menkes and Lexchin, "Letter."
34 Styrap, *A Code of Medical Ethics*.
35 Spence, "Bad Medicine," 526.
36 Harrison and Kouzel, "Cyberchondria."
37 Husain and Spence, "Can Healthy People Benefit from Health Apps?"
38 Feke, "Dr. Google."
39 Avery, Ghandi, and Keating, "The 'Dr Google' Phenomenon."
40 Goyder, McPherson, and Glasziou, "Self Diagnosis."
41 Rugby is the national sport in New Zealand, where I come from. To a New Zealand reader, this example is as familiar as the expression "three strikes and you're out!" to North Americans, baseball fans or not.
42 The rules have recently changed to ensure that the on-field referee controls the game. He now must posit his on-field assessment, and ask for confirmation or not of that decision. "I see a try (touchdown). Can you confirm

that this is the case?" Here, as in medicine, the change in rule attempts to locate authority in one specific site.

43 Gualtieri, "The Doctor as the Second Opinion."
44 Blaxter, "Diagnosis as Category and Process."
45 Brown, "Naming and Framing."
46 See, for example, my own work, Jutel, "Sociology of Diagnosis"; and Jutel and Nettleton, "Towards a Sociology of Diagnosis"; but also McGann and Hutson, *Sociology of Diagnosis*; and Smith-Morris, *Diagnostic Controversy*.
47 Zola, *Socio-Medical Inquiries*.
48 Whooley, *Knowledge in the Time of Cholera*.
49 See, for example, Dumit, "Illnesses You Have to Fight to Get"; Nettleton et al., "Enigmatic Illness"; and Malterud, "[Subjective Symptoms without Objective Findings]."

3 "The Expertness of His Healer"

1 Hippocrates, "Prognosis."
2 Schofield, *Unconscious Therapeutics*, 113.
3 Whooley, *Knowledge in the Time of Cholera*.
4 Doctors have long been advisers on childhood, old age, pregnancy, and so on.
5 And, in particular, the employ of power is harder to recognize as such when we think about our contemporary setting, usually in more practical than critical terms.
6 Beauchamps, "Informed Consent."
7 Emanuel and Emanuel, "Four Models of the Physician-Patient Relationship."
8 Cathell, *The Physician Himself*, 50.
9 Cathwell, 49.
10 I discovered no writings on this subject from this era by female doctors, so am resorting to the gender-specific pronoun for this part of the chapter.
11 Harrison, *Medical Ethics*.
12 Harrison, 10.
13 Richardson, "Telling the Truth to Patients."
14 Richardson, 436.
15 Richardson, 435
16 Schofield, *Unconscious Therapeutics*, 109.
17 Schofield, 95–6.
18 Richardson, "Telling the Truth to Patients."
19 Collins, "Should Doctors Tell the Truth?" 320.

20 Seelig, "Should Cancer Victims Be Told the Truth?" 43.
21 Balch, "Some Psychological Observations by the Surgeon," 131.
22 Whooley, *Knowledge in the Time of Cholera*.
23 National Library of Medicine, s.v. "Truth Disclosure," accessed October 12, 2018, https://www.ncbi.nlm.nih.gov/mesh/?term=truth-disclosure.
24 Brown, *Health: Five Lay Sermons to Working People*.
25 Brown, 33.
26 Hooker, *Physician and Patient*, 381.
27 Hooker, 50.
28 Cabot, "'Justifiable' Lying," 146.
29 Crenner, *Private Practice in the Early Twentieth-Century Medical Office*, 219.
30 Crenner.
31 Hallenbeck, "A Surgeon's View."
32 Litin, "Should the Cancer Patient Be Told?"; Rynearson, "An Internist's View"; Westberg, "Advice to the Family."
33 Litin et al., "Panel Discussion."
34 Mitchell, *Doctor and Patient*, 47–8.
35 Mitchell, 47.
36 Palfrey, *The Art of Medical Treatment*, x.
37 Palfrey, 20.
38 Riggs, "The Significance of Illness," 119.
39 Riggs, 120.
40 Sperry, *The Ethical Basis of Medical Practice*, 987.
41 Davidson, "What to Tell the Gravely Ill Patient," 116.
42 Little, *Doctors and the Public*, 8.
43 American Medical Association, *Code of Ethics*, 2.
44 Saundby, *Medical Ethics*, 105.
45 Little, *Doctors and the Public*, 8.
46 Palfrey, *The Art of Medical Treatment*, 20–1.
47 Johnson, *The True Physician*, 127–8.
48 Martin, *The Woman in the Body*.
49 Sanders, *Every Patient Tells a Story*, xiii.
50 Osler, *The Principles and Practice of Medicine*, 7.
51 Sanders, 8.
52 Mukherjee, *The Emperor of All Maladies*.
53 Fludernik, *Towards a "Natural" Narratology*.
54 Mukherjee, 152–3.
55 Mukherjee, 307.
56 Mukherjee, 307.

57 Mukherjee, 400.
58 Mukherjee, 400.
59 Mukherjee, 400.
60 Mukherjee, 400.
61 Srivastava, *Tell Me the Truth*.
62 Srivastava, 2.
63 Srivastava, 227.
64 Srivastava, 216.
65 Srivastava, 38.
66 Srivastava, 39.
67 Srivastava, 293.
68 Srivastava, 306.
69 Srivastava, 306.
70 Foucault described the political economy of truth as being "characterized by five important traits. Truth is centred on the form of scientific discourse and the institutions which produce it; it is subject to constant economic and political incitement (the demand for truth, as much for economic production as for political power); it is the object, under diverse forms, of immense diffusion and consumption (circulating through apparatuses of education and information whose extent is relatively broad in the social body, notwithstanding certain strict limitations); it is produced and transmitted under the control, dominant if not exclusive, of a few great political and economic apparatuses (university, army, writing, media); lastly, it is the issue of a whole political debate and social confrontation ('ideological' struggles)" (Foucault, *Power/Knowledge*, 131).
71 Freidson, *Profession of Medicine*, 244.
72 Crenner, *Private Practice in the Early Twentieth-Century Medical Office*.
73 Balint, *The Doctor, His Patient and the Illness*, 18.
74 Balint, 18.
75 Balint, 25.
76 Surbone, "Telling the Truth," 57.
77 Cathell, *The Physician Himself*, 107.
78 Mütter, *Charge to the Graduates of Jefferson Medical College of Philadelphia*, 12.
79 Blaxter, "The Case of the Vanishing Patient?" 776.

4 "The News Is Not Altogether Comforting"

1 McEwan, *Saturday*.
2 McEwan, 91

 3 McEwan, 94; this quotation was to become my epigraph.
 4 McEwan, 94.
 5 McEwan, 95.
 6 Funder, *All That I Am*.
 7 Funder, 7.
 8 Funder, 8.
 9 Funder, 9.
10 Funder, 353.
11 Funder, 259.
12 Funder, 294.
13 Funder, 346.
14 Funder, 37.
15 Morpurgo, *Alone on a Wide, Wide Sea*.
16 Morpurgo, 12.
17 Morpurgo, 11.
18 Morpurgo, 14.
19 Morpurgo, 194–5.
20 Morpurgo, 105.
21 Hailey, *The Final Diagnosis*.
22 Hailey, 28.
23 Hailey, 49.
24 Hailey, 72.
25 Hailey, 499.
26 Obreht, *The Tiger's Wife*.
27 Obreht, 30.
28 Obreht, 68.
29 Obreht, 182.
30 Obreht, 299.
31 Obreht, 311.
32 Hill, *The Various Haunts of Men*.
33 Thompson, *Helsinki White*.
34 Kemelman, *Wednesday the Rabbi Got Wet*.
35 Kemelman, 65–6.
36 McWatt, *Vital Signs*.
37 Robinson, *Gilead*.
38 Robinson, 5.
39 Banks, *Complicity*.
40 Zerubavel, "Generally Speaking."
41 Kemelman, *Wednesday the Rabbi Got Wet*.

42 Banks, *Complicity*, 311.
43 Banks, "A Personal Statement."
44 Frank, "The Rhetoric of Self-Change."

5 Breaking Bad

1 Abbott, *The Cambridge Introduction to Narrative*.
2 Bordwell, *Poetics of Cinema*.
3 Bordwell.
4 Bordwell.
5 Gilligan, *Breaking Bad*.
6 Lilti, *Médecin de campagne*.
7 Gilligan, *Breaking Bad*.
8 Tzanelli and Yar, "*Breaking Bad*, Making Good"; and Pierson, "*Breaking Bad*."
9 Frow, *Genre*, 2.
10 Brooks, *The Melodramatic Imagination*.
11 Elsaesser, "Tales of Sound and Fury."
12 Gledhill, "The Melodramatic Filed."
13 Eyre, *Iris*.
14 Hiller, *Love Story*.
15 Claudel, *I've Loved You So Long*.
16 Glatzer and Westmoreland, *Still Alice*.
17 Hayward, "Melodrama and Women's Films."
18 Arcand, *Decline of the American Empire*.
19 Zilberman, *A Late Quartet*.
20 Mulvey, "Notes on Sirk and Melodrama."
21 Mike Nichols, *Wit*.
22 Rimmon-Kenan, "Margaret Edson's *Wit*."
23 Rimmon-Kenan, 352.
24 Klaver, "A Mind-Body-Flesh Problem," 662.
25 Nichols, "Angels in America."
26 Soderbergh, "Side Effects."
27 DiFrancesco, "Facing the Specter of Immigration in Biutiful."
28 Balint, *The Doctor, His Patient and the Illness*.
29 Varda, *Cléo de 5 à 7*.
30 Mouton, "From Feminine Masquerade to Flâneuse."
31 Hitchcock, *Psycho*.
32 Claudel, *I've Loved You So Long*.

33 Hankir et al., "Cinematherapy and Film"; Datta, "Madness and the Movies"; and Wilson et al., "Madness at the Movies."

6 A Picture Paints a Thousand Words

1 Williams, "Graphic Medicine."
2 Balint, *The Doctor, His Patient and the Illness*.
3 Jutel, "Classification, Disease, and Diagnosis."
4 Dumit, "Illnesses You Have to Fight to Get."
5 Gardner, "Let's Send That to the Lab."
6 Frank, *The Wounded Storyteller*.
7 Frank, 5–6.
8 Grootens-Wiegers et al., "Comic Strips Help Children Understand."
9 Thomas and Ashwal, *Iggy and the Inhalers*; and Green and Myers, "Graphic Medicine."
10 Krakow, "Graphic Narratives and Cancer Prevention."
11 Green, "Teaching with Comics."

7 The Intellectual Documentary

1 Fleischman, "A Linguist Reflects."
2 Fleischman, 10.
3 Frank, "The Rhetoric of Self-Change," 39.
4 Frank, *The Wounded Storyteller*, 17.
5 Frank, "The Standpoint of Storyteller," 355.
6 Couser, "Body Language."
7 Kalanithi, *When Breath Becomes Air*.
8 Boesky, *The Story Within*. Readers interested in the illness narrative should imperatively read Art Frank's *The Wounded Storyteller*, Arthur Kleinman's *The Illness Narratives*, and Ann Jurecic's *Illness as Narrative*.
9 Blaxter, "The Case of the Vanishing Patient?"
10 Carel, "With Bated Breath."
11 Stoddard Holmes, "Pink Ribbons and Public Private Parts."
12 Blaxter, "Diagnosis as Category and Process."
13 Daly, Conrad, Prior et al, Ettorre, Barker, Frank, and so on, in Blaxter, "The Case of the Vanishing Patient?"
14 For example, Cussins, Mol, Latour and Kelly, Radstake in Blaxter, "The Case of the Vanishing Patient?"
15 Blaxter, "Diagnosis as Category and Process," 768.
16 Blaxter, "Diagnosis as Category and Process," 774.

17 Blaxter, "Diagnosis as Category and Process," 776.
18 Fleischman, 4.
19 Fleischman, 4.
20 Fleischman, 5.
21 Fleischman, 12.
22 Fleischman, 6.
23 Fleischman, 7.
24 Fleischman, 8.
25 Sontag, *Illness as Metaphor*.
26 Sontag, 4.
27 Zerubavel, "Lumping and Splitting."
28 Davison, Smith, and Frankel, "Lay Epidemiology and the Prevention Paradox."
29 Fleischman, 24.
30 Carel, "With Bated Breath."
31 Carel, *Illness: The Cry of the Flesh*.
32 Carel, "With Bated Breath," 60.
33 Carel, "With Bated Breath," 61. I must editorialize here that this comment is in relation to Carel's own physical illness. Other diagnoses, particularly psychiatric ones, but also some physical ones (think diseases related to sexual function) may induce, rather than release, the sense of shame.
34 Carel, "With Bated Breath," 61.
35 When I called my dad in the United States the moment I learned of his serious and ultimately life-shortening diagnosis, his "philosophical" reply was, "Well, there is nothing certain in life but death and taxes!"
36 Carel, "Should I Fear My Death?"
37 Carel, "Should I Fear My Death?" 117.
38 Carel, *Illness: The Cry of the Flesh*, 120.
39 Carel, *Illness: The Cry of the Flesh*, 148.
40 Carel, Illness: The Cry of the Flesh, 17.
41 Stoddard Holmes, "Pink Ribbons and Public Private Parts."
42 Stoddard Holmes, 481.
43 Stoddard Holmes, 482.
44 Stoddard Holmes, 481.
45 Stoddard Holmes, 492.
46 Vertinsky, *The Eternally Wounded Woman*.
47 Lorde, *The Cancer Journals*, 7.
48 Lorde, 8.
49 Frank, "Tricksters and Truth Tellers," 191.
50 Frank, 190.

51 Charon, *Narrative Medicine*, 65–6.

52 Charon, 65.

53 Charon, 9–10.

54 Glaser and Strauss, *Awareness of Dying*, 8–9.

55 Jutel, "Beyond the Sociology of Diagnosis."

56 Zerubavel, "Generally Speaking."

57 Zerubavel, 133.

58 Zerubavel, 136.

59 Coser, *Masters of Sociological Thought*, quoted in Zerubavel, "Generally Speaking," 136.

60 Douglas, *Purity and Danger*, 94.

61 Oakley, *Fracture*.

62 Ettorre, "Making Sense of my Illness Journey."

63 Caplan, "Chronic Fatigue Syndrome."

64 Carver, "What the Doctor Said."

8 What's There to Tell?

1 Whedon, *The Avengers*.

2 Whedon, *The Avengers*.

3 Differential diagnosis is the process of differentiating between potential candidate diagnoses to arrive upon the final diagnosis.

4 Whedon identified as the goal of the diagnosis: "I needed to get Banner [Hulk's human name] from the horror of what he had done ... into, you know, a place where he was prepared to go back into that [Hulk] state. He needs somebody who will just accept him" (Cassidy, "The Avengers").

5 Wilkins, "No Hugging, Some Learning."

6 Wilkins.

7 Morrison, Quitely, and Grant, *All-Star Superman*.

8 Lorde, 52.

9 Lorde, 53.

10 Alan Barry in Surbone, "Telling the Truth to Patients"

11 A point that Havi Carel maintained in her philosophical illness narrative where she posited that the diagnostic moment could be one of opportunity, as opposed to trauma.

12 Whooley, *Knowledge in the Time of Cholera*.

13 Williams, *The Bad Doctor*.

14 Thomas and Ashwal, *Iggy and the Inhalers*.

15 Brody, "'My Story Is Broken.'"

16 Balint, *The Doctor, His Patient and the Illness*.

17 Goyal, "Narration in Medicine."
18 Spencer, "Narrative Medicine."
19 Charon, 224–5.
20 White and Epston. *Narrative Means to Therapeutic Ends.*
21 Lutz, "The Oldest Library Motto"; White and Epston, *Narrative Means to Therapeutic Ends.*
22 Johnson, *The True Physician*, 146–7.
23 McAlister, "Bibliotherapy."
24 Frank, "Tricksters and Truth Tellers."
25 Haddock, *Da Vinci's Inquest.*
26 Obreht, *The Tiger's Wife.*
27 Shore, *House, MD.*
28 Nichols, *Wit.*
29 Hill, *The Various Haunts of Men.*
30 Zilberman, *A Late Quartet.*
31 Blaxter, "The Case of the Vanishing Patient?"
32 L'Engle, *A Wrinkle in Time.*
33 Abbott, *The Cambridge Introduction to Narrative.*

References

Abbott, H. Porter. *The Cambridge Introduction to Narrative*. 2nd ed. Cambridge Introductions to Literature. Cambridge, UK: Cambridge University Press, 2008.

American Medical Association. *Code of Ethics of the American Medical Association*. Chicago, IL: American Medical Association, 1847. https://collections .nlm.nih.gov/bookviewer?PID=nlm:nlmuid-63310420R-bk.

Arcand, Denys, dir. *Decline of the American Empire*. Montreal, QC: Corporation Image M & M, 1986.

Arnold, Thomas. *On the Divisions and Mutual Relations of Knowledge: A Lecture Read before the Rugby Literary and Scientific Society, April 7, 1835*. Rugby, UK: Combe and Crossley, 1839.

Aronowitz, R. "Framing Disease: An Underappreciated Mechanism for the Social Patterning of Health." *Social Science & Medicine* 67, no. 1 (2008): 1–9.

Avery, N., J. Ghandi, and J. Keating. "The 'Dr Google' Phenomenon – Missed Appendicitis." *The New Zealand Medical Journal* 125, no. 1367 (2012): 135–7.

Bainbridge, William Seaman. "The Cancer Campaign Quaternary: The Problem, the Public, the Patient, the Physician." *American Journal of Surgery* 31, no. 6 (1917): 162–7.

Balch, Franklin G. "Some Psychological Observations by the Surgeon." In *Physician and Patient: Personal Care*, edited by L. Eugene Emerson, 122–42. Cambridge, MA: Harvard University Press, 1929.

Balint, Michael. *The Doctor, His Patient and the Illness*. 2nd ed. Kent, UK: Pitman Medical, 1964.

Banks, Iain. "A Personal Statement from Iain Banks." April 3, 2013. https://
www.iain-banks.net/2013/04/03/a-personal-statement-from-iain-banks/.
– *Complicity*. 1st ed. New York: Doubleday, 1995.
Beauchamps, Tom L. "Informed Consent: Its History, Meaning, and Present
Challenges." *Cambridge Quarterly of Healthcare Ethics* 20, no. 4 (2011): 515–23.
Bettevy, F., C. Dufranc, and G. Hofmann. "Les enjeux du dispositif d'annonce:
le point de vue de la Ligue nationale contre le cancer." *Oncologie* 8 (2006):
515–17.
Blaxter, Mildred. "Diagnosis as Category and Process: The Case of Alcohol-
ism." *Social Science and Medicine* 12 (1978): 9–17.
– "Life Narratives, Health and Identity." In *Identity and Health*, edited by Da-
vid Kelleher and Gerard Leavey, 170–99. New York: Routledge, 2004.
– "The Case of the Vanishing Patient? Image and Experience." *Sociology of
Health and Illness* 31, no. 5 (2009): 762–78.
Boesky, Amy, ed. *The Story Within: Personal Essays on Genetics and Identity*.
Baltimore: Johns Hopkins University Press, 2014.
Bordwell, David. *Poetics of Cinema*. New York: Routledge, 2008.
Bowker, Geoffrey C. "The History of Information Infrastructures: The Case
of the International Classification of Diseases." *Information Processing and
Management* 32, no. 1 (1996): 49–61.
Bowker, Geoffrey C., and Susan Leigh Star. *Sorting Things Out: Classification
and Its Consequences*. Inside Technology. Cambridge, MA: MIT Press, 1999.
Brackenbury, Henry Britten. *Patient and Doctor*. London: Hodder and Stough-
ton, 1935.
Bresalier, Michael. "'A Most Protean Disease': Aligning Medical Knowledge of Modern Influenza, 1890–1914." *Medical History* 56, no. 4 (2012):
481–510.
Brody, Howard. "'My Story Is Broken; Can You Help Me Fix It?': Medical Eth-
ics and the Joint Construction of Narrative." *Literature and Medicine* 13, no. 1
(1994): 79–92.
Brooks, Peter. *The Melodramatic Imagination: Balzac, Henry James, Melodrama,
and the Mode of Excess*. Columbia University Press Morningside ed. New
York: Columbia University Press, 1985.
Broughton, Arthur. *Observations on the Influenza, or Epidemic Catarrh; as It Ap-
peared in Bristol and Its Environs, During the Months of May and June, 1782. To
Which Is Added, a Meteorological Journal*. 1782.
Brown, John. *Health: Five Lay Sermons to Working People*. New York: Robert
Carter & Brothers, 1862.
Brown, Phil. "Naming and Framing: The Social Construction of Diagnosis and
Illness." *Journal of Health and Social Behavior Health Module* (1995): 34–52.

Brown, Phil. "The Name Game: Toward a Sociology of Diagnosis." *The Journal of Mind and Behaviour* 11, no. 3–4 (1990): 385–406.

Broyard, Anatole. "Doctor, Talk to Me." In *On Doctoring*, edited by Richard Reynolds and John Stone, 175–81. New York: Simon and Schuster, 1995.

Budd, Alice, Lenee Blanton, Lisa Groshkopf, Angela Campbell, Vivien Dugan, David E. Wentworth, and Lynette Brammer. "Influenza." In *Manual for the Surveillance of Vaccine-Preventable Diseases*, edited by Sandra W. Roush, Linda M. Baldy, and Mary Ann Kirkconnell, chapter 6. Atlanta, CA: Centers for Disease Control and Prevention, 2008.

Cabot, Richard C. "'Justifiable' Lying." *The Journal of Education* 69, no. 6 (1909): 145–6.

Caplan, Paula J. "Chronic Fatigue Syndrome." *Women & Therapy* 23, no. 1 (2001): 23–43.

Carel, Havi. "Should I Fear My Death?" In *BoB Lectures*, edited by Havi Carel. Bristol, UK: Bristol University, 2016.

– "With Bated Breath: Diagnosis of Respiratory Illness." *Perspectives in Biology and Medicine* 58, no. 1 (2015): 53–65.

– *Illness: The Cry of the Flesh*. Stocksfield, UK: Acumen Press, 2008.

Carrat, Fabrice, Elisabeta Vergu, Neil M Ferguson, Magali Lemaitre, Simon Cauchemez, Steve Leach, and Alain-Jacques Valleron. "Time Lines of Infection and Disease in Human Influenza: A Review of Volunteer Challenge Studies." *American Journal of Epidemiology* 167, no. 7 (2008): 775–85.

Carver, Raymond. "What the Doctor Said." In *A New Path to the Waterfall*, 113. New York: Atlantic Monthly Press, 1989.

Cassidy, Mark. "The Avengers: Joss Whedon on Harry Dean Stanton's Cameo; Why He Was Chosen for His Scene with Mark Ruffalo." ComicBookMovie. com. March 5, 2012. https://www.comicbookmovie.com/avengers/the-avengers-joss-whedon-on-harry-dean-stantons-cameo-why-he-was-chosen-a59032.

Cathell, Daniel Webster. *The Physician Himself and What He Should Add to His Scientific Acquirements in Order to Secure Success*. 5th ed. Baltimore: Cushings & Bailey, 1885.

Centers for Disease Control and Prevention. "Update: Novel Influenza A (H1N1) Virus Infections – Worldwide, May 6, 2009." In *Morbidity and Mortality Weekly Report*, 453–8: Centers for Disease Control and Prevention, 2009.

– "Avian Influenza A Virus Infections in Humans." Last modified April 18, 2017. https://www.cdc.gov/flu/avian/gen-info/avian-flu-humans.htm.

– "Outbreak of Swine-Origin Influenza a (H1N1) Virus Infection – Mexico, March–April 2009." Last modified April 30, 2009. https://www.cdc.gov/mmwr/preview/mmwrhtml/mm58d0430a2.htm.

Charon, Rita. *Narrative Medicine: Honoring the Stories of Illness*. Oxford: Oxford University Press, 2006.

Charon, Rita, and Martha Montello. *Stories Matter: The Role of Narrative in Medical Ethics*. Reflective Bioethics. New York: Routledge, 2002.

Claudel, Philippe, dir. *I've Loved You So Long*. France: UGC Distribution, 2008.

Collins, Joseph. "Should Doctors Tell the Truth?" *Harper's Monthly Magazine* 155 (1927): 320–6.

"Commerce without Conscience." *The British Medical Journal* 2, no. 3994 (24 July 1937): 178–9.

Couser, G. Thomas. "Body Language: Illness, Disability, and Life Writing." *Life Writing* 13, no. 1 (2016): 3–10.

Crenner, Christopher. *Private Practice in the Early Twentieth-Century Medical Office of Dr. Richard Cabot*. Baltimore: Johns Hopkins University Press, 2005.

Croskerry, Pat. "Achieving Quality in Clinical Decision Making: Cognitive Strategies and Detection of Bias." *Academic Emergency Medicine* 9, no. 11 (2002): 1184–205.

Datta, Vivek. "Madness and the Movies: An Undergraduate Module for Medical Students." *International Review of Psychiatry* 21, no. 3 (2009): 261–6.

Davidson, Maurice. "What to Tell the Gravely Ill Patient, or One Who Has to Undergo a Serious Operation." In *Medical Ethics: A Guide to Students and Practitioners*, edited by Maurice Davidson, 109–19. London: Lloyd-Luke (Medical Books) Ltd., 1957.

Davison, Charlie, George Davey Smith, and Stephen Frankel. "Lay Epidemiology and the Prevention Paradox: The Implications of Coronary Candidacy for Health Education." *Sociology of Health and Illness* 13, no. 1 (1991): 1–19.

De Shazer, Mary, and Anita Helle. "Theorizing Breast Cancer: Narrative, Politics, Memory." *Tulsa Studies in Women's Literature* 32, no. 2 (2013): 7–23.

DiFrancesco, Maria. "Facing the Specter of Immigration in *Biutiful*." *Symposium: A Quarterly Journal in Modern Literatures* 69, no. 1 (2015): 25–37.

Doherty-Torstrick, Emily R., Kate E. Walton, and Brian A. Fallon. "Cyberchondria: Parsing Health Anxiety from Online Behavior." *Psychosomatics* 57, no. 4 (2016): 390–400.

Douglas, Mary. *Purity and Danger*. London: Routledge and Kegan Paul, 1966.

Dumit, Joseph. "Illnesses You Have to Fight to Get: Facts as Forces in Uncertain, Emergent Illnesses." *Social Science & Medicine* 62, no. 3 (2006): 577–90.

Elsaesser, Thomas. "Tales of Sound and Fury: Observations on the Family Melodrama." In *A Reader on Film and Television Melodrama*, edited by Marcia Landy, 68–91. Detroit: Wayne State University Press, 1971.

Emanuel, Ezekiel J., and Linda L. Emanuel. "Four Models of the Physician-Patient Relationship." *Journal of the American Medical Association* 267, no. 16 (1992): 2221–6.

Epidemic and Pandemic Alert and Response. "Addressing Ethical Issues in Pandemic Influenza Planning: Discussion Papers." Geneva: World Health Organization, 2008.

Ettorre, Elizabeth. "Making Sense of My Illness Journey from Thyrotoxicosis to Health: An Autoethnography." *Auto / Biography* 14, no. 2 (2006): 153–75.

Eyre, Richard, dir. *Iris*. London: British Broadcasting Corporation, 2001.

Fadiman, Anne. *The Spirit Catches You and You Fall Down: A Hmong Child, Her American Doctors, and the Collision of Two Cultures*. 1st ed. New York: Farrar, Straus, and Giroux, 1997.

Feke, Tanya. "Dr Google Should Be Sued for Malpractice. Here's Why." KevinMD.com. August 9, 2015. https://www.kevinmd.com/blog/2015/08/dr-google-should-be-sued-for-malpractice-heres-why.html.

Fergus, Thomas A., and Sara L. Dolan. "Problematic Internet Use and Internet Searches for Medical Information: The Role of Health Anxiety." *Cyberpsychology, Behavior, and Social Networking* 17, no. 12 (2014): 761–5.

Fleischman, Suzanne. "I Am … , I Have … , I Suffer From … A Linguist Reflects on the Language of Illness and Disease." *Journal of Medical Humanities* 20, no. 1 (1999): 1–31.

Fludernik, Monika. *Towards a "Natural" Narratology*. London; New York: Routledge, 1996.

Foucault, Michel. *Power/Knowledge: Selected Interviews and Other Writings, 1972–1977*. Edited by Colin Gordon. 1st American ed. New York: Pantheon Books, 1980.

Frank, Arthur W. "Just Listening: Narrative and Deep Illness." *Families, Systems and Health* 16, no. 3 (1998): 197.

– "Tricksters and Truth Tellers: Narrating Illness in an Age of Authenticity and Appropriation." *Literature and Medicine* 28, no. 2 (2009): 185–99.

– "The Rhetoric of Self-Change: Illness Experience as Narrative." *The Sociological Quarterly* 34, no. 1 (1993): 39–52.

– "The Standpoint of Storyteller." *Qualitative Health Research* 10, no. 3 (2000): 354–65.

– *The Wounded Storyteller: Body, Illness and Ethics*. Chicago: University of Chicago Press, 1995.

Freidson, Eliot. *Profession of Medicine: A Study of the Sociology of Applied Knowledge*. 4th ed. New York: Dodd, Mead & Company, 1972.

Frenkel, Moshe, Joan C. Engebretson, Sky Gross, Noemi E. Peterson, Ariela
    Popper Giveon, Kenneth Sapire, and Doron Hermoni. "Exceptional Patients
    and Communication in Cancer Care – Are We Missing Another Survival
    Factor?" *Supportive Care in Cancer* 24, no. 10 (2016): 4249–55.
Frow, John. *Genre*. 2nd ed. The New Critical Idiom. New York: Routledge,
    2015.
Funder, Anna. *All That I Am: A Novel*. 1st US ed. New York: Harper, 2011.
Gardner, John. "Let's Send That to the Lab: Technology and Diagnosis." In
    Social Issues in Diagnosis: An Introduction for Students and Clinicians, edited
    by Annemarie Goldstein Jutel and Kevin Dew, 155–64. Baltimore: Johns
    Hopkins University Press, 2014.
Gelsomini, Mirko, Franca Garzotto, Daniele Montesano, and Daniele Oc-
    chiuto. "Wildcard: A Wearable Virtual Reality Storytelling Tool for Children
    with Intellectual Developmental Disability." *Conference of the IEEE Engineer-
    ing in Medicine and Biology Society* (2016): 5188–91.
Gersuny, Robert. *Doctor and Patient: Hints to Both*. Bristol, UK: John Wright &
    Co, 1889.
Gilligan, Vince, dir. *Breaking Bad*. Culver City, CA: Sony Pictures Television, 2008.
Gilman, Charlotte Perkins. *The Yellow Wall Paper*. Boston: Small, Maynard &
    Company, 1899.
Glaser, Barney G., and Anselm L. Strauss. *Awareness of Dying*. Chicago: Aldine
    Publishing Company, 1968.
Glatzer, Richard, and Wash Westmoreland, dirs. *Still Alice*. New York: Sony
    Pictures Classics, 2014.
Gledhill, Christine. "The Melodramatic Filed: An Investigation." In *Home Is
    Where the Heart Is: Studies in the Melodrama and the Woman's Film*, edited by
    Christine Gledhill, 5–39. London: British Film Institute, 1987.
Global Influenza Surveillance and Response System (GISRS). "Standardiza-
    tion of Terminology of the Pandemic A(H1N1)2009 Virus." World Health
    Organization, 2011. http://www.who.int/influenza/gisrs_laboratory/
    terminology_ah1n1pdm09/en/.
Goyal, Rishi. "Narration in Medicine." In *The Living Handbook of Narratol-
    ogy*, edited by Peter Hühn et al. Hamburg: Hamburg University. Last
    revised August 21, 2013. http://www.lhn.uni-hamburg.de/article/
    narration-medicine.
Goyder, Clare, Ann McPherson, and Paul Glasziou. "Self Diagnosis." *BMJ* 339
    (2009): b4418. https://doi.org/10.1136/bmj.b4418.
Green, Michael J. "Teaching with Comics: A Course for Fourth-Year Medical
    Students." *Journal of Medical Humanities* 34, no. 4 (2013): 471–6.

Green, Michael J., and Kimberly R. Myers. "Graphic Medicine: Use of Comics in Medical Education and Patient Care." *BMJ* 340 (2010): c863.

Grootens-Wiegers, Petronella, Martine C. de Vries, Mara M. van Beusekom, Laura van Dijck, and Jos M. van den Broek. "Comic Strips Help Children Understand Medical Research: Targeting the Informed Consent Procedure to Children's Needs." *Patient Education and Counseling* 98, no. 4 (2015): 518–24.

Gualtieri, Lisa Neal. "The Doctor as the Second Opinion and the Internet as the First." In *CHI '09 Extended Abstracts on Human Factors in Computing Systems*, 2489–98. Boston: Association for Computing Machinery, 2009.

Hacking, Ian. "Inaugural Lecture: Chair of Philosophy and History of Scientific Concepts at the Collège De France, 16 January 2001." *Economy and Society* 31, no. 1 (2001): 1–14.

Haddock, Chris, dir. *Da Vinci's Inquest*. Toronto: Canadian Broadcasting Corporation, 1998–2006.

Hadra, Berthold E. *The Public and the Doctor. By a Regular Physician*. Dallas: Franklin Press, 1902.

Hailey, Arthur. *The Final Diagnosis, a Novel*. 1st ed. Anstey, Leicestershire, UK: F.A. Thorpe (Publishing) Ltd, 1959.

Hallenbeck, George, A. "A Surgeon's View." *Staff Meetings of the Mayo Clinic* 35, no. 10 (1960): 243–47.

Hankir, Ahmed, David Holloway, Rashid Zaman, and Mark Agius. "Cinematherapy and Film as an Educational Tool in Undergraduate Psychiatry Teaching: A Case Report and Review of the Literature." *Psychiatria Danubina* 27 Suppl 1 (2015): S136–42.

Hanne, Michael, and Susan J. Hawken. "Metaphors for Illness in Contemporary Media." *Medical Humanities* 33, no. 2 (2007): 93–9.

Harrison, John P. *Medical Ethics: A Lecture Delivered 23 December 1843 before the Ohio Medical Lyceum*. Cincinnati: Enquirer and Message Print, 1844.

Harrison, Kathryn L., and Omar Kouzel. "Cyberchondria." *Student BMJ* 17 (2009).

Hayward, Susan. "Melodrama and Women's Films." In *Cinema Studies: The Key Concepts*, 213–26. London: Routledge, 2000.

Hemingway, Ernest. "A Day's Wait." *Literary Cavalcade* 51, no. 6 (1999/1936): 18–20.

Hill, Amelia, and Robin McKie. "Ten Years On: It's Time to Count the Costs of the Viagra Revolution." *The Guardian*, February 25, 2008. https://www.theguardian.com/theobserver/2008/feb/24/controversiesinscience.

Hill, Susan. *The Various Haunts of Men*. London: Vintage, 2005.

Hiller, Arthur, dir. *Love Story*. Hollywood: Paramount Pictures, 1970.

Hippocrates. "Prognosis." In *Hippocratic Writings*, edited by G.E.R. Lloyd, 170–85. London: Penguin, 1983.

Hitchcock, Alfred, dir. *Psycho*. Hollywood: Paramount Pictures, 1960.

Hooker, Worthington. *Physician & Patient: Or, a Practical View of the Mutual Duties, Relations & Interests of the Medical Profession & the Community. From the Text of Worthington Hooker*, edited by Edward Bentley. London: Edward Bentley, 1850.

Houlihan, Catherine F., Sanjay Patel, David A. Price, Manoj Valappil, and Uli Schwab. "Life Threatening Infections Labelled Swine Flu." *BMJ* 340 (2010): c137.

Houston, Thomas K., Gemmae M. Fix, Stephanie L. Shimada, Judith A. Long, Howard S. Gordon, Charlene Pope, Julie Volkman, Jeroan J. Allison, Kathryn DeLaughter, Michelle Orner, and Barbara G. Bokhour. "African American Veterans Storytelling: A Multisite Randomized Trial to Improve Hypertension." *Medical Care* 55 Suppl 9 Suppl 2 (2017): S50-s58.

Hughes-Jones, Philip. "Study of Influenza." *The British Medical Journal* 4, no. 5885 (20 October 1973): 178, https://doi.org/10.1136/bmj.4.5885.178-a.

Hunsaker Hawkins, Anne. "Pathography: Patient Narratives of Illness." *The Western Journal of Medicine* 171, no. 2 (1999): 127–9.

Husain, Iltifat, and Des Spence. "Can Healthy People Benefit from Health Apps?" *BMJ* 350, no. 8004 (2015): 16–17. https://doi.org/10.1136/bmj.h1887.

ICD Update Platform. *Influenza, Avian Flu, Flu Pandemic 2009, Other Epidemiological Important Influenzas*. Geneva: World Health Organization, 2010.

Johnson, Wingate Memory. *The True Physician; the Modern "Doctor of the Old School."* New York: Macmillan Company, 1936.

Judicial Watch. "Illegal Aliens Spread Swine Flu in Us." April 30, 2009. https://www.judicialwatch.org/blog/2009/04/illegal-aliens-spread-swine-flu-u-s/.

Jutel, Annemarie. "Beyond the Sociology of Diagnosis." *Sociology Compass* 9, no. 9 (2015): 841–52.

– "Classification, Disease, and Diagnosis." *Perspectives in Biology and Medicine* 54, no. 2 (2011): 189–205.

– "The Emergence of Overweight as a Disease Category: Measuring up Normality." *Social Science and Medicine* 63, no. 9 (2006): 2268–76.

– "Self-Diagnosis: A Discursive Systematic Review of the Medical Literature." *Journal of Participatory Medicine* 2, no. 15 (2010): e8.

– "Sociology of Diagnosis: A Preliminary Review." *Sociology of Health and Illness* 31, no. 2 (2009): 278–99.

– "When Pigs Could Fly: Influenza and the Elusive Nature of Diagnosis." *Perspectives in Biology and Medicine* 56, no. 4 (2013): 513–29.

Jutel, Annemarie Goldstein. *Putting a Name to It: Diagnosis in Contemporary Society*. Baltimore: Johns Hopkins University Press, 2011.

Jutel, Annemarie Goldstein, Michael G. Baker, James Stanley, Q. Sue Huang, and Don Bandaranayake. "Self-Diagnosis of Influenza During a Pandemic: A Cross-Sectional Survey." *BMJ Open* 1, no. 2 (January 2011).

Jutel, Annemarie Goldstein, and Elizabeth Banister. "'I Was Pretty Sure I Had the Flu': Qualitative Description of Confirmed-Influenza Symptoms." *Social Science & Medicine* 99 (2013): 49–55.

Jutel, Annemarie Goldstein, and Barbara Mintzes. "Female Sexual Dysfunction: Medicalizing Desire." In *Routledge International Handbook of Critical Mental Health*, edited by Bruce Cohen, 162–8. New York: Routledge, 2017.

Jutel, Annemarie Goldstein, and Sarah Nettleton. "Towards a Sociology of Diagnosis: Reflections and Opportunities." *Social Science & Medicine*, Special Issue (2011): 793–800.

Kalanithi, Paul. *When Breath Becomes Air*. 1st ed. New York: Random House, 2016.

Keall, Chris. "New Zealand Added to Google Swine Flu Map." *New Zealand Business Review*. Accessed 31 October 2016. https://www.nbr.co.nz/article/new-zealand-added-google-swine-flu-map-101628.

Keith, Robert D. *Clinical Case-Taking*. London: H.K. Lewis & Co. Ltd., 1918.

Kemelman, Harry. *Wednesday the Rabbi Got Wet*. Greenwich, CT: Fawcett Crest, 1976.

Kim, Hyosun. "Trouble Spots in Online Direct-to-Consumer Prescription Drug Promotion: A Content Analysis of FDA Warning Letters." *International Journal of Health Policy and Management* 4, no. 12 (2015): 813–21.

Klaver, Elizabeth. "A Mind-Body-Flesh Problem: The Case of Margaret Edson's Wit." *Contemporary Literature* 45, no. 4 (2006): 659–83.

Klawiter, Maren. "Breast Cancer in Two Regimes: The Impact of Social Movements on Illness Experience." *Sociology of Health and Illness* 26, no. 6 (September 2004): 845–74. https://doi.org/10.1111/j.1467-9566.2004.421_1.x.

Krakow, Melinda. "Graphic Narratives and Cancer Prevention: A Case Study of an American Cancer Society Comic Book." *Health Communication* 32, no. 5 (May 2017): 525–8.

Krecke, Albert. *The Doctor and His Patients*, edited by Fritz Lange. London: Kogan Paul, Trench, Trubner, 1934.

Lacey, Nick. *Image and Representation: Key Concepts in Media Studies*. New York: Palgrave, 1998.

Lapham, Roger, F. *Disease and the Man*. New York: Oxford University Press, 1937.

Latour, Bruno. "Why Has Critique Run out of Steam? From Matters of Fact to Matters of Concern." *Critical Inquiry* 30, no. 2 (2004): 225–48.

Leder, Drew. "Clinical Interpretation: The Hermeneutics of Medicine." *Theoretical Medicine* 11 (1990): 9–24.

– *The Absent Body*. Chicago: University of Chicago Press, 1990.

Leibmann-Smith, Richard. "Swine Flu over the Cuckoo's Nest." *New Yorker*, May 31, 1976, 31.

Lemon, George William. *English Etymology; or a Derivative Dictionary of the English Language in Two Alphabets*. London: G. Robinson, 1701.

L'Engle, Madeleine. *A Wrinkle in Time*. New York: Farrar, Straus, and Giroux, 1962.

Lilti, Thomas. *Médecin de campagne*. Paris: Le Pacte, 2016.

Litin, Edward M. "Should the Cancer Patient Be Told?" *Postgraduate Medicine* 28, no. 5 (November 1960): 470–5.

Litin, Edward M., Gunnar B. Stickler, Edward H. Rynearson, George A. Hallenbeck, Malcolm B. Dockerty, Clifford F. Gastineau, Howard P. Rome, Gershom J. Thompson, and Frank J. Heck. "Panel Discussion." *Staff Meetings of the Mayo Clinic* 35, no. 10 (1960): 251–7.

Little, E. Graham. *Doctors and the Public: An Address Delivered at the Opening of the Medical Session at St. George's Medical School on October 1st, 1926*. Foxton, UK: Burlington Press, 1926.

Locock, Louise, Sarah Nettleton, Susan Kirkpatrick, Sara Ryan, and Sue Ziebland. "'I Knew before I Was Told': Breaches, Cues and Clues in the Diagnostic Assemblage." *Social Science & Medicine* 154 (2016): 85–92.

Lorde, Audré. *The Cancer Journals*. San Francisco: Aunt Lute Books, 1980.

Louriz, Maha, Chafiq Mahraoui, Abderrahim Azzouzi, Mohamed Taoufiq El Fassy Fihri, Amine Ali Zeggwagh, Khalid Abidi, Driss Ferhati, et al. "Clinical Features of the Initial Cases of 2009 Pandemic Influenza A (H1N1) Virus Infection in an University Hospital of Morocco." *International Archives of Medicine* 3 (2010): 26.

Lund, Charles, C. "The Doctor, the Patient and the Truth." *Annals of Internal Medicine* 24, no. 6 (1946): 955–60.

Lupton, Deborah. "Consumerism, Reflexivity and the Medical Encounter." *Social Science and Medicine* 45, no. 3 (1997): 373–81.

Lutz, Cora E. "The Oldest Library Motto." *The Library Quarterly: Information, Community, Policy* 48, no. 1 (1978): 36–9.

Mackey, Tim K. "Digital Direct-to-Consumer Advertising: A Perfect Storm of Rapid Evolution and Stagnant Regulation: Comment on 'Trouble Spots in Online Direct-to-Consumer Prescription Drug Promotion: A Content

Analysis of FDA Warning Letters.'" *International Journal of Health Policy Management* 5, no. 4 (2016): 271–5.

Malterud, K. "[Subjective Symptoms without Objective Findings – A Challenge for Theory and Practice of General Medicine]." *Ugeskr Laeger* 163, no. 48 (2001): 6729–34.

Martin, Emily. *The Woman in the Body: A Cultural Analysis of Reproduction.* Boston: Beacon Press, 1992.

McAlister, Clifton. "Bibliotherapy." *The American Journal of Nursing* 50, no. 6 (1950): 356–7.

McEwan, Ian. *Saturday.* 1st ed. New York: Doubleday, 2005.

McGann, P. J., and David J. Hutson, eds. *Sociology of Diagnosis.* Bingley, UK: Emerald, 2011.

McNeil, Donald J. "The Ethics of Hunting Down 'Patient Zero.'" *New York Times*, October 30, 2016. https://www.nytimes.com/2016/10/30/sunday-review/the-ethics-of-hunting-down-patient-zero.html?_r=0.

McWatt, Tessa. *Vital Signs: A Novel.* Toronto: Random House Canada, 2011.

Menkes, David B., and Joel Lexchin. "Letter: Skilled Use of the Media by Vested Interests to Promote Drugs and Other Health Products." *BMJ* 352 (2016): i1179. https://doi.org/10.1136/bmj.i1179.

Metzl, Jonathan. *The Protest Psychosis: How Schizophrenia Became a Black Disease.* Boston: Beacon Press, 2009.

Mitchell, S. Weir. *Conduct of the Medical Life: Addressed to the Students of the University of Pennsylvania and the Jefferson Medical College.* Philadelphia: University of Pennsylvania Press, 1893.

– *Doctor and Patient.* Philadelphia: J. B. Lippincott Company, 1888.

Morpurgo, Michael. *Alone on a Wide, Wide Sea.* London: Harper Collins Children's Books, 2006.

Morrison, Grant, Frank Quitely, and Jamie Grant. *All-Star Superman.* Superman, edited by Jeb Woodard. Burbank, CA: DC Comics, 2011.

Mouton, Janice. "From Feminine Masquerade to Flaneuse: Agnès Varda's Cléo in the City." *Cinema Journal* 40, no. 2 (2001): 3–16.

Mukherjee, Siddhartha. *The Emperor of All Maladies: A Biography of Cancer.* Large print ed. Waterville, ME: Thorndike Press, 2010.

Mulvey, Laura. "Notes on Sirk and Melodrama." In *Home Is Where the Heart Is: Studies in Melodrama and the Woman's Film*, edited by Christine Gledhill, 75–9. London: British Film Institute, 1987.

Mütter, Thomas, D. *Charge to the Graduates of Jefferson Medical College of Philadelphia.* Philadelphia: TK and PG Collins, Printers, 1851.

Nerlich, Brigitte, and Christopher Halliday. "Avian Flu: The Creation of Expectations in the Interplay between Science and the Media." *Sociology of Health and Illness* 29, no. 1 (January 2007): 46–65.

Nettleton, Sarah, Lisa O'Malley, Ian Watt, and Philip Duffey. "Enigmatic Illness: Narratives of Patients Who Live with Medically Unexplained Symptoms." *Social Theory & Health* 2 (2004): 47–66.

Nichols, Mike, dir. *Angels in America*. New York: HBO, 2003.

– *Wit*. 2001; New York: HBO, 2001.

Nicoll, Angus. "Planning for Uncertainty: A European Approach to Informing Responses to the Severity of Influenza Epidemics and Pandemics." *Bulletin of the World Health Organization* 89 (2011): 542–4.

Oakley, Ann. *Fracture: Adventures of a Broken Body*. Bristol, UK: Policy Press, 2007.

Obreht, Téa. *The Tiger's Wife*. London, UK: Phoenix, 2011.

Osler, William. *The Principles and Practice of Medicine: Designed for the Use of Practitioners and Students of Medicine*. New York: D. Appleton and Co, 1892.

Palfrey, Francis W. *The Art of Medical Treatment: With Reference Both to the Patient and His Friends*. Philadelphia: W.B. Saunders Company, 1925.

Parsons, Talcott. "Definitions of Health and Illness in the Light of American Values and Social Structure." In *Patients, Physicians and Illness: Behavioral Science and Medicine*, edited by E. Gartly Jaco, 165–87. Glencoe, IL: The Free Press, 1958.

Pierson, David P. *"Breaking Bad": Critical Essays on the Contexts, Politics, Style, and Reception of the Television Series*. Lanham, MD: Lexington Books, 2014.

Plato. *Plato in Twelve Volumes*, translated by Harold N. Fowler. Vol. 9. Cambridge, MA: Harvard University Press, 1925.

Potter, C. W. "A History of Influenza." *Journal of Applied Microbiology* 91, no. 4 (2001): 572–9.

Prior, Lindsay, Meirion R. Evans, and Hayley Prout. "Talking About Colds and Flu: The Lay Diagnosis of Two Common Illnesses among Older British People." *Social Science & Medicine* 73, no. 6 (2011): 922–8.

Reiser, Stanley J. "Words as Scalpels: Transmitting Evidence in the Clinical Dialogue." *Annals of Internal Medicine* 92, no. 6 (1980): 837–42.

Richardson, Maurice H. "Telling the Truth to Patients with Serious or Hopeless Disease." *St. Paul Medical Journal* 11 (1909): 429–52.

Riggs, Austen Fox. "The Significance of Illness." In *Physician and Patient: Personal Care*, edited by L. Eugene Emerson, 100–21. Cambridge, MA: Harvard University Press, 1929.

Rimmon-Kenan, Shlomith. "Margaret Edson's *Wit* and the Art of Analogy." *Style* 40, no. 4 (2006): 346–56.

Robinson, Maralyn. *Gilead*. New York: Farrar, Straus and Giroux, 2004.

Rosenberg, Charles, E. "Contested Boundaries: Psychiatry, Disease and Diagnosis." *Perspectives in Biology and Medicine* 49, no. 3 (2006): 407–24.

Rynearson, Edward, H. "An Internist's View." *Staff Meetings of the Mayo Clinic* 11 (May 1960): 240–3.

Sachs, Bernard. "Be an Optimist." *Journal of Mount Sinai Hospital* 8 (1942): 323–5.

Sanders, Lisa. *Every Patient Tells a Story: Medical Mysteries and the Art of Diagnosis.* 1st ed. New York: Broadway Books, 2009.

Saundby, Robert. *Medical Ethics: A Guide to Professional Conduct.* London: Charles Griffin & Company, 1907.

Schofield, Alfred T. *Unconscious Therapeutics; or, the Personality of the Physician.* Philadelphia: P. Blakiston's, 1906.

Schuster, David G. "Personalizing Illness and Modernity: S. Weir Mitchell, Literary Women, and Neurasthenia, 1870–1914." *Bulletin of the History of Medicine* 79, no. 4 (Winter 2005): 695–722.

Seelig, M. G. "Should Cancer Victims Be Told the Truth?" *Journal of, the Missouri State Medical Association* 40 (1943): 33–5.

Shore, David, dir. *House, M.D.* New York: NBC Universal Television Distribution, 2004–2012.

Shortland, H. Brandt. *Findings of Coroner H. B. Shortland.* Auckland: Coroner's Court, 2011.

Smith-Morris, Carolyn. *Diagnostic Controversy: Cultural Perspectives on Competing Knowledge in Healthcare.* Routledge Studies in Anthropology. New York: Routledge, Taylor & Francis Group, 2016.

Soderbergh, Steven, dir. *Side Effects.* Los Angeles, CA: Open Road Films, 2013.

Sontag, Susan. *Illness as Metaphor.* New York: Farrar, Straus and Giroux, 1978.

Spence, Des. "Bad Medicine: The Worried Hell." *British Journal of General Practice* 66, no. 651 (2016): 526.

Spencer, Danielle. "Narrative Medicine." In *The Routledge Companion to the Philosophy of Medicine,* edited by Miriam Solomon, Jeremy R. Simon, and Harold Kincaid, 372–82. New York: Routledge, 2017.

Sperry, Willard, L. *The Ethical Basis of Medical Practice.* New York: Paul B. Hoeber, Inc., 1950.

Srivastava, Ranjana. *Tell Me the Truth: Conversations with My Patients About Life and Death.* Melbourne: Penguin Books, 2010.

Star, Susan Leigh, and James R. Griesemer. "Institutional Ecology, 'Translations' and Boundary Objects: Amateurs and Professionals in Berkeley's Museum of Vertebrate Zoology, 1907–39." *Social Studies of Science* 19, no. 3 (1989): 387–420.

Stearns, Peter. *Fat History: Bodies and Beauty in the Modern West.* New York: New York University Press, 1997.

Stephenson, Niamh, and Michelle Jamieson. "Securitising Health: Australian Newspaper Coverage of Pandemic Influenza." *Sociology of Health and Illness* 31, no. 4 (May 2009): 525–39.

Stoddard Holmes, Martha. "Pink Ribbons and Public Private Parts." *Literature and Medicine* 25, no. 2 (2006): 475–501.

Styrap, Jukes. *A Code of Medical Ethics: With Remarks on the Duties of the Practitioners to Their Patients, and the Obligation of Patients to Their Medical Advisers.* London: J & A Churchill, 1878.

Surbone, Antonella. "Telling the Truth to Patients with Cancer: What Is the Truth?" *The Lancet Oncology* 7, no. 11 (2006): 944–50.

Surbone, Antonella. "Truth Telling." *Annals of the New York Academy of Sciences* 913, no. 1 (2000): 52–62.

Taubenberger, Jeffery K., Johan V. Hultin, and David M. Morens. "Discovery and Characterization of the 1918 Pandemic Influenza Virus in Historical Context." *Antiviral Therapy* 12, no. 4 Pt B (2007): 581–91.

Te Poel, Fam, Susanne E. Baumgartner, Tilo Hartmann, and Martin Tanis. "The Curious Case of Cyberchondria: A Longitudinal Study on the Reciprocal Relationship between Health Anxiety and Online Health Information Seeking." *Journal of Anxiety Disorders* 43 (October 2016): 32–40.

Thomas, Alex, and Gary Ashwal. *Iggy and the Inhalers.* Santa Monica, CA: Booster Shot Media, 2015.

Thompson, James. *Helsinki White: An Inspector Vaara Novel.* New York: G. P. Putnam's Sons, 2012.

Tielman, Myrthe L., Mark A. Neerincx, Rafael Bidarra, Ben Kybartas, and Willem-Paul Brinkman. "A Therapy System for Post-Traumatic Stress Disorder Using a Virtual Agent and Virtual Storytelling to Reconstruct Traumatic Memories." *Journal of Medical Systems* 41, no. 8 (2017): 125.

Tognotti, Eugenia. "Scientific Triumphalism and Learning from Facts: Bacteriology and the 'Spanish Flu' Challenge of 1918." *Social History of Medicine: The Journal of the Society for the Social History of Medicine / SSHM* 16, no. 1 (April 2003): 97–110.

Trilla, Anthony, Guillem Trilla, and Carolyn Daer. "The 1918 'Spanish Flu' in Spain." *Clinical Infectious Diseases* 47, no. 5 (2008): 668–73.

Tzanelli, Rodanthi, and Majid Yar. "*Breaking Bad*, Making Good: Notes on a Televisual Tourist Industry." *Mobilities* 11, no. 2 (2016): 188–206.

Varda, Agnès, dir. *Cléo de 5 À 7.* Paris: Athos Filmes, 1962.

Vertinsky, Patricia A. *The Eternally Wounded Woman: Women, Doctors, and Exercise in the Late Nineteenth Century.* Champaign: University of Illinois Press, 1994.

Vickers, Lucy. "College Caught in Flu Scare." *Stuff.* May 8, 2009. http://www.stuff.co.nz/auckland/2366791/College-caught-in-flu-scare.

Vorhaus, Martin G. *The Changing Patient-Doctor Relationship*. New York: Horizon Press, 1957.

Wailoo, Keith. *Drawing Blood: Technology and Disease Identity in Twentieth-Century America*. Baltimore: Johns Hopkins University Press, 1997.

Westberg, Granger, C. "Advice to the Family on Being Given the Diagnosis of Cancer." *The Medical Clinics of North America* 42, no. 2 (1958): 563–8.

Whedon, Joss, dir. *The Avengers*. Hollywood: Marvel Studios, Paramount Pictures, 2012.

Whooley, Owen. *Knowledge in the Time of Cholera: The Struggle over American Medicine in the Nineteenth Century*. Chicago: University of Chicago Press, 2013.

Wilkins, Damien. "No Hugging, Some Learning: Writing and Personal Change." In *The Fuse Box: Essays on Writing from Victoria University's International Institute of Modern Letters*, edited by Emily Perkins and Chris Price, 101–21. Wellington, Australia: Victoria University Press, 2017.

Williams, Ian C. *The Bad Doctor*. Graphic Medicine. University Park: The Pennsylvania State University Press, 2015.

Williams, Ian C. "Graphic Medicine: Comics as Medical Narrative." *Medical Humanities* 38, no. 1 (2012): 21–7.

Willis, Thomas. *The Remaining Medical Works of That Famous and Renowned Physician Dr Thomas Willis*. London: T. Dring, C. Harper, J. Leigh and S. Martyn, 1681.

Wilson, Nick, Deb Heath, Tim Heath, Peter Gallagher, and Mark Huthwaite. "Madness at the Movies: Prioritised Movies for Self-Directed Learning by Medical Students." *Australas Psychiatry* 22, no. 5 (2014): 450–3.

Wooldridge, Frosty. "Swine Flu-Immigration, Death and Disease … And Consequences for Americas." Rense. April 27, 2009. https://rense.com/general85/sw.htm.

World Health Organization. "WHO Issues Best Practices for Naming New Human Infectious Diseases." News release, May 8, 2015. http://www.who.int/mediacentre/news/notes/2015/naming-new-diseases/en/.

Zerubavel, Eviatar. "Generally Speaking: The Logic and Mechanics of Social Pattern Analysis." *Sociological Forum* 22, no. 2 (2007): 131–45.

– "Lumping and Splitting: Notes on Social Classification." *Sociological Forum* 11, no. 3 (1996): 421–33.

Zilberman, Yaron, dir. *A Late Quartet*. New York: Opening Night Productions, 2012.

Zola, Irving Kenneth. *Socio-Medical Inquiries: Recollections, Reflections, and Reconsiderations*. Philadelphia: Temple University Press, 1983.

Index